# OPHTHALMIC NURSING

## SECOND EDITION

## Rosalind Stollery

SRN SCM FETC DipN (Lond) OND Cert Ed
Teaching Fellow
University of Southampton School of Nursing and Midwifery

D0353500

**Blackwell**
Science

053937

610.73 677

© 1997 by Blackwell Science Ltd, a
Blackwell Publishing Company
Editorial Offices:
Osney Mead, Oxford OX2 0EL, UK
   Tel: +44 (0)1865 206206
Blackwell Science, Inc., 350 Main Street,
Malden, MA 02148-5018, USA
   Tel: +1 781 388 8250
Iowa State Press, a Blackwell Publishing
Company, 2121 State Avenue, Ames, Iowa
50014-8300, USA
   Tel: +1 515 292 0140
Blackwell Publishing Asia Pty Ltd, 550
Swanston Street, Carlton South, Melbourne,
Victoria 3053, Australia
   Tel: +61 (0)3 9347 0300
Blackwell Wissenschafts Verlag,
Kurfürstendamm 57, 10707 Berlin, Germany
   Tel: +49 (0)30 32 79 060

First published 1987
Second edition 1997
Reprinted 1999, 2001, 2003

Library of Congress
Cataloging-in-Publication Data
Stollery, Rosalind
    Ophthalmic nursing/Rosalind Stollery.
  —2nd ed.
    Includes bibliographical references and
index.
    ISBN 0-632-03996-5 (alk. paper)
    1. Ophthalmic nursing.   I. Title.
    [DNLM: 1. Eye Diseases—nursing.
WY 158 S875o 1997]
RE88.S76   1997
610.73'677—dc20                     96-28897
                                                           CIP

ISBN 0-632-03996-5

A catalogue record for this title is available
from the British Library

Set in 10/12 pt Palatino
by DP Photosetting, Aylesbury, Bucks
Printed and bound in India
by Thomson press (India).

For further information on
Blackwell Publishing, visit our website:
www.blackwellpublishing.com

€33.66

# Contents

# Foreword

by Heather Waterman *PhD, BSc (Hons), RGN, OND, DipN*
Chair, RCN Ophthalmic Nursing Forum

In approximately one fifth of ophthalmic units/hospitals there is none or only one nurse holding ophthalmic qualifications (Waterman *et al.* 1995). Larger hospitals and units are well endowed with ophthalmic nurses; unfortunately this is not the case everywhere. More ophthalmic nurses are required if patients in smaller units are to receive care comparable to those in bigger ophthalmic units.

It is obvious that nurses with knowledge and skills gained from an ophthalmic course will be in a far better position to understand the reasons behind certain approaches to care and consequently offer more rigorous care to patients. They will, for example, perceive the necessity for positioning patients after vitrectomy surgery. Their grasp of the anatomy and physiology of the eye and orbit, and ophthalmic treatment will be such that they will be able to provide comprehensive and thorough care, particularly in the education of patients. They are likely to be prepared to educate other groups of nurses who come across patients with ophthalmic conditions, including diabetes nurse specialists and practice nurses, and to treat developments and changes in care and the service as opportunities to improve patient care and advance practice. It is false economy not to educate nurses in ophthalmics for their is evidence to suggest that those with ophthalmic qualifications are able to expand their practice further to function in complimentary medical positions, for example, as nurse practitioners in eye casualty departments. Ophthalmic nurses do not replace doctors (as one doctor may for another) but because they view patients 'holistically', they are concerned to perform the medical task and to educate and support patients as well. Nurses without an ophthalmic qualification are unlikely to aspire to be nurse specialists or practitioners. Ophthalmic trained nurses are good value for money and are worth investing in financially.

The publication of the second edition of *Ophthalmic Nursing* is timely bearing in mind the need to educate nurses in ophthalmics. This book is a valuable resource and quick reference text, which informs in a straightforward manner. It is user-friendly and will encourage non-ophthalmic nurses to read on and learn more. Examples of patient information leaflets are presented clearly and offer very useful guides to the education of

patients. The second edition updates the reader in advances in ophthalmic technology and care since the first edition was published in 1987.

## Reference

Waterman H., Hope K., Beed P., Clayton E., McQueen L., Owen C., Stott M. and
    Studley M., (1995) The nature of ophthalmic services, and the education and
    qualifications of nurses: a national survey. *Journal of Advanced Nursing,* **22,**
    914–20.

# Preface

There have been many advances in ophthalmic nursing since the first edition of this book in 1987. Microsurgery, increased use of the laser, advanced investigation techniques, new drugs and the change in the emphasis on delivery of care from inpatient to a day case/outpatient basis have all made an impact on the care the nurse must give the ophthalmic patient. In this new edition all of these aspects have been taken into account with emphasis being given to patient education and to the assessment skills now required of nurses as they have less contact time with patients.

However, the book remains a fundamental text aimed primarily at those nurses commencing their ophthalmic experience or as an *aide-mémoire* for those with some ophthalmic knowledge. It is a useful text for those taking ophthalmic nursing courses, for teachers, for trained and untrained nurses. It may also be useful for nurses who may come across patients with ophthalmic problems in areas such as care of the elderly, accident and emergency and industry.

In order to recognise the diploma/degree level of ophthalmic courses some references have been included, covering research and other sources of information for readers to follow up if they wish. It is hoped that the inclusion of references will not impede the easy flow of the text. It is not intended to be an academic essay! The chapters are well illustrated with relevant diagrams and photographs.

In this edition the first two chapters describe the patients presenting with ophthalmic conditions and varying visual impairments and the nurse's responsibility to those patients in the ward and day case areas and the casualty, outpatient and operating departments. The chapter on nursing procedures now includes the rationale for such skills. Trauma has been highlighted as a new key chapter.

A brief description of the eye and its blood and nerve supply is given in Chapter 4, although each structure of the eye is described more thoroughly in subsequent chapters. These chapters give details of diseases related to each structure. The nursing action to be taken in response to the needs of the patient suffering from these specific conditions is described in order that the nurse can plan the patient's care.

The psychological and physical effects of removal of an eye and the subsequent nursing care are the subjects of Chapter 15. The final chapter on ophthalmic drugs in common use gives the usual doses, side effects and any special points about each drug.

There is a useful Index of Symptoms describing which structure and related condition may be involved with each ophthalmic symptom.

The medical and physiological influence in the text is deliberate which may be criticised by some nurses. Unless practitioners have a sound knowledge and understanding of the structures of the eye, and the conditions that affect it, they will be unable to plan, deliver and evaluate effective patient care.

Finally, for the sake of ease and clarity, the nurse is referred to as 'she' and the patient as 'he' with no discrimination intended.

*R. Stollery*

# Acknowledgements

I would like to thank my family, friends and colleagues at the University of Southampton School of Nursing and Midwifery and Southampton Eye Unit for their help and encouragement in writing this edition. I am particularly grateful to Southampton Eye Unit for the use of the material within their patient information leaflets.

Special thanks must go to Krys Coster and Anne Millo, senior orthoptists, for their invaluable assistance with the section on squints, to Sisters Jagir Sahota and Gillian Pead for their help with the section on theatre nursing, Sue Wakelin, pharmacist, Polly Tadevossian, social worker and to Mr Peng Khaw for his guidance and for allowing me to use some of his photographs.

The illustrations have come from various sources and in addition to those acknowledged within the text, I also wish to acknowledge P.D. Trevor-Roper and P.V. Curran's *The Eye and its Disorders* (2nd edn), P.D. Trevor-Roper's *Lecture Notes on Ophthalmology* (7th edn) and *Pocket Consultant Ophthalmology* (2nd edn) all published by Blackwell Science. If I have failed to mention a specific source it is hoped that the author/ publisher will accept this blanket acknowledgement and my gratitude.

# 1 The Ophthalmic Patient

## 1.1 INTRODUCTION

The ophthalmic patient may be of any age, from a few days to over 100 years old. Ophthalmic conditions affect all age groups, though the highest proportion of patients are the elderly.

Most infants and children will have parents who wish to be involved in their child's care. The child whose parents are either unable or unwilling to become involved will need the extra care and attention of a nurse to reassure him in unfamiliar and possibly frightening surroundings.

The ophthalmic patient may have other diseases such as diabetes, ankylosing spondylitis and arthritis, as these have ocular manifestations. He may also suffer from unrelated diseases.

The ophthalmic patient will arrive at the eye hospital or unit either as a referral to the outpatient department or as a casualty, where many are self-referred and may not be 'emergencies' as such. They will present with a variety of conditions from a lump on the lid to sudden visual loss or severe trauma.

Most people will be anxious on a first visit to a hospital. Even for the elderly, but otherwise fit, person it might be his first experience of a hospital. Those arriving following trauma will be in varying degrees of shock depending on the accident. They and their relatives may be very anxious. Something which seems fairly minor to the nurse with ophthalmic knowledge may, to a layman, appear serious and be thought to threaten sight.

Many people have a fear of their eyes being touched, making examination difficult. Some feel faint, or do faint, while certain procedures, such as removal of a foreign body, are being performed.

There are some old wives' tales about the eye. One of the commonest appears to be the fact that the eye can be removed from the socket for examination and treatment, and be replaced afterwards. This kind of false knowledge does not help the patient's frame of mind.

Each person will arrive at the hospital with his own individual personality and past experience to colour any attitude towards the eye condition. Some will be stoical, others extremely agitated. Those with chronic

1

or recurrent eye conditions may become more used to visiting the eye hospital. Most patients having ophthalmic surgery are either outpatients, day cases or overnight-stay patients. This means they have a very short time to adjust to the hospital setting and have little time to ask questions that may be initially forgotten in the midst of all the activity. They may feel reluctant to express minor concerns when there appears to be little contact time with nurses.

The actual visual impairment experienced by the patient will vary with the eye condition. With many conditions there is no, or only slight, visual impairment. Others cause gross visual loss which may have occurred suddenly or gradually over the years. This visual loss may be untreatable and permanent, may be progressive, or sight may be restored. Some patients will have only one eye affected, others both eyes, probably to different degrees. Some will have blurred vision, some will be able to make out only movements. Others will be able to differentiate only between light and dark, or will see nothing at all. Some will have lost their central vision, others their peripheral vision. Some patients will see better in bright light than dim light, and vice versa. Some degrees of visual loss can be very upsetting to the patient and prove to be a severe impairment to daily living. All patients experiencing severe visual loss will require practical and emotional help in coming to terms with it, regardless of the cause and the course it has taken.

## 1.2   REGISTRATION FOR THE BLIND AND PARTIALLY SIGHTED

Research carried out by the Royal National Institute for the Blind (RNIB) (Bruce *et al.* 1991) suggested that three-quarters of people eligible for registration are not in fact registered.

### 1.2.1   Blind register

The statutory definition for the purpose of registration as a blind person under the National Assistance Act 1948 is that the person 'is so blind as to be unable to perform any work for which eyesight is essential'. This refers to any form of employment, not only that which the patient formerly followed. It also only takes into account visual impairment, other bodily or mental infirmities being disregarded. People with a visual acuity of less than 3/60 on the Snellen Chart (see Section 3.2.2) or with a visual acuity of 6/60 but with a marked peripheral field defect will be eligible for registration.

### 1.2.2   Partially sighted register

There is no statutory definition of partial sight but a person who does not qualify to be registered as blind but nevertheless is substantially visually impaired can be registered as partially sighted. Those people with 3/60 to 6/60 vision and full peripheral field, those with vision up to 3/60 with moderate visual field contraction, opacities in the media, aphakia and those with 6/18 or better visual acuity but marked field loss can be included on this register.

## 1.3   ASSISTANCE AND REHABILITATION

The National Assistance Act 1948 directs all local authorities to compile a register of blind and partially sighted people residing in their area and to provide advice, guidance and services to enable these people and their families to maintain their independence and live as full a life as possible.

Registration is voluntary. People can choose to register but if they do register they can have their names removed from the register at any time should they decide. The local authority has the responsibility to review the register regularly and to update the circumstances of the people on it. Local authorities must offer services to all those identified as visually impaired whether they choose to register or not. However, registration is necessary to qualify for financial benefits and for help from the many voluntary organisations. Registration is a good guide as to whether a person is coming to terms with their sight loss.

The process of registration starts with the ophthalmologist certifying on a form numbered BD8 in England and Wales, BP1 in Scotland and A655 in Northern Ireland that a person is eligible for either blind or partially sighted registration. The person signs this form agreeing for information on the form to be shared with their local Social Services, General Practitioner and the Department of Population Census which maintains records of all those opting to share this information.

The Social Services Department has the responsibility to register people. Some social services departments have delegated this task to their local voluntary organisation which deals with the blind and partially sighted people within their area. The role of the social worker is that of counsellor. They provide support and information about the services available. This includes entitlement to benefits and referral to other statutory bodies involved with retraining, special needs education for those of school and college age, rehabilitation, employment, social, leisure and recreational activities and introduction to self-help groups.

## 1.4   VOLUNTARY ORGANISATIONS

There are a number of voluntary organisations that work with the visually impaired. Most local areas or counties have their own organisations. These are established to provide aids and social contact for the visually impaired. Many local authorities have an arrangement with voluntary organisations to provide services to facilitate independent living such as talking or tactile watches and clocks to alarms that sound when rained upon so that the washing can be brought in. The increase in technology has resulted in equipment being available, for example, to enlarge print on to a TV screen, to convert the written word into Braille or to use voice synthesisers.

Local voluntary organisations are often centres of social contact for the visually impaired and their carers.

# 2  The Ophthalmic Nurse

## 2.1  INTRODUCTION

The ophthalmic nurse must naturally possess all the qualities required of a nurse working in any speciality or environment. There are, though, some characteristics that are more important to a nurse specialising in the diseases and conditions of the eye.

The eye is very delicate and sensitive. Most of the patients the nurse will attend to will have varying degrees of pain or discomfort in or around the eye. Therefore she must be extremely gentle with her hands and in her manner in order to allay any fears the patient may have about his eyes being touched.

The eye is small and there is not much room for manoeuvre around it when performing manual nursing procedures. The nurse therefore needs to be manually dexterous. She also needs to have the best possible vision when performing nursing procedures, and is doing the patient no justice by being vain and not wearing glasses for close work should these be required.

As ophthalmic patients can be from any age group, the nurse needs to be familiar with the special requirements of all ages, those of the very young and the old in particular.

The nurse must be thoughtful in her approach to the visually impaired person. She must use touch, introduce herself, indicate when she is leaving and never shout. There is a great temptation to assume that a person who is visually impaired is also hard of hearing.

The nurse must always bear in mind that there is an individual person behind the eyes that are being treated, and care for each patient as a whole, unique person.

## 2.2  ASSESSMENT OF PATIENTS

Most ophthalmic patients receive treatment as outpatients, day cases or, if hospitalised, tend to spend a minimum of time actually in hospital. This means that the nurse no longer has the luxury of time in which to get to

5

know the patient and be able to assess his needs and therefore must employ succinct assessment skills in order to carry out an effective assessment.

Assessment is said to be the most important interaction nurses have with patients (Barker 1985) and MacLeod-Clarke (1988) contends that to assess an individual effectively requires excellent communication skills. The ophthalmic nurse must, therefore, use verbal and non-verbal skills appropriately. Open-ended questions yield more information and an appropriate tone and pitch of voice should be employed. She must be aware of the effects of eye contact, facial expression, posture, gestures and touch on the patients, remembering that non-verbal communication apart from touch is not appropriate to the visually impaired. It is also useful to employ minimal counselling skills described by Burnard (1991) as the use of listening, silence, attention and paraphrasing. The ophthalmic nurse also needs to be very observant.

## 2.3   PATIENT INFORMATION AND TEACHING

The Patient's Charter (DoH 1995) requires that patients are given information about their conditions and treatments. It is well recognised by nurses that giving information relieves anxiety and aids recovery. Not only do patients and carers need to know what is wrong with them and what the management is, but the majority will want to know why. Having an understanding of the rationale behind treatment will aid compliance and enable the patient to be actively involved. Patients and carers need information at all stages of management. Research has shown that patients benefit from preoperative teaching programmes (Allen *et al.* 1992; Latham *et al.* 1992).

Nurses may be the only professional to impart the necessary information. Even when the doctor has given information, the patients tend to see the nurse as the one to explain that information (Milburn *et al.* 1995). The ophthalmic nurse must, therefore, be in possession of sound knowledge in order to impart accurate information. She also needs time and the ability to use communication skills, mentioned above, appropriately. The nurse needs to assess how much information the patient needs and to what depth and whether to use lay or professional terminology. The ophthalmic nurse needs to be able to impart information to all age groups. As the majority are elderly, she needs a special understanding of this age group. Although the senses are often reduced due to the ageing process, Potter (1994) claims that the elderly are able to learn about their health. Visually impaired elderly with a hearing loss are a challenge to the ophthalmic nurse, especially as loss of both of these senses may cause confusion.

In addition to providing information on the various conditions and

## PATIENT INFORMATION LEAFLET No. 1

# HOW TO USE YOUR EYE DROPS

Read the instructions carefully. Treat only the eye stated. If you have any difficulty it may be better to get someone to put the drops in for you.

(1)   Wash your hands.

(2)   Tilt your head backwards and look towards the ceiling. Gently pull down the lower lid to form a pouch.

(3)   Drop the prescribed number of drops (usually one) into the pouch. Do not touch the eyelid or eye with the dropper.

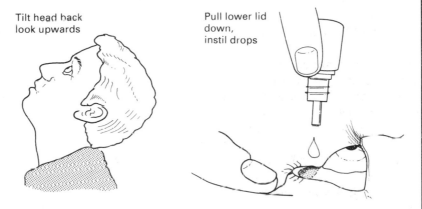

Tilt head back
look upwards

Pull lower lid
down,
instil drops

(4)   Close your eyes (do not rub them) and blink several times.

(5)   With your fingers, apply gentle pressure to the bridge of your nose for a few minutes. This prevents the drops being drained from your eye.

(6)   Remove any excess solution by wiping your eye lashes with a clean tisue.

(7)   Replace the cap of the eye drops immediately after use.

If the drops cause blurred vision do not drive or operate machinery until your vision has cleared.

Discard the drops in accordance with the instructions on the label.

ALWAYS leave at least 5–10 minutes between instilling eye preparations.

When instilling eye drops and eye ointment at the same time of day ALWAYS instil the eye drops FIRST.

their treatment, the nurse also needs to instruct the patient or carer in practical skills which need to be carried out at home such as instilling drops (see Patient Information Leaflet No. 1), lid hygiene or inserting shells. The patient or carer will need to have time to practice these skills following instruction from the nurse. It is vital that the nurse assesses their competence, which needs to be satisfactory, if compliance is to be achieved. Compliance can be a problem for a number of reasons (Williams 1993; Patel & Speath 1995). These can include forgetfulness, lack of motivation, side effects of the drops and the frequency of their instillation. Physical problems such as hand tremor and weakness or arthritis may be overcome by the use of devices to help in the delivery of drops.

Teaching is another area that has been affected by the shortened contact time between nurse and patient. The actual organisation of when and where to perform this teaching is often difficult. Verbal information and instruction must be backed up with the written word (see examples of Patient Information Leaflets and Advice Sheets in the following text), both of which must be clear, unambiguous and appropriate for the individual.

The patient's need for information and the nurse's role to give it are vitally important and, in order to save tedious repetition in the following text, it will be assumed under each eye condition, that this is carried out.

Above all, the ophthalmic nurse needs to be a knowledgeable, competent practitioner who instils confidence in the patients with whom she has contact.

## 2.4  PROFESSIONAL ISSUES

The ophthalmic nurse of today needs to be research aware and should be encouraged to become involved in research studies or research-related activities especially as there has been little nursing research in the speciality so far. However, it could be said that it is more important that the ophthalmic nurse has a general and comprehensive grasp of research issues and is able to read and respond to relevant research findings (Robinson 1994).

Nurses are being encouraged to be reflective in their practice and the ophthalmic nurse is no exception. Reflection allows time for nurses to ponder on or in their practice and discover ways to improve their performance. Reflection is encouraged as it fills the theory/practice gap in nursing (Conway 1994).

The UKCC *Scope of Professional Practice* (UKCC 1992) urges nurses to expand their scope of practice and ophthalmic nurses are in an ideal position to do so as technology advances in the ophthalmic world. However, nurses must not take on these roles at the expense of their nursing duties. They must also have the required underpinning knowledge otherwise they may become mere technicians.

Ophthalmic nurses should take note of the statement in *A Strategy for Nursing* (DoH 1989) that states 'all practitioners should develop skills in and use every opportunity for health promotion'. This would include informing people of accident prevention and screening for diseases such as open-angle glaucoma.

Ophthalmic nurses are required to be involved with quality audit and standard setting. A nurse without ophthalmic knowledge and understanding of the patient's needs will not be able to set or audit appropriate standards which Tingle (1992) suggests should be 'realistic, reasonable and relevant'.

## 2.5  THE NURSE IN THE OUTPATIENT DEPARTMENT

The outpatient department is the portal into the hospital or unit for the majority of patients attending with eye conditions and may be the only department they visit. The nurse working there should therefore be a good advertisement for the whole hospital or unit.

Outpatient departments are always busy and there seems to be no answer to the problem of waiting time. There are ways that the nurse can alleviate the frustrations and boredom experienced due to the waiting. She can inform the patient approximately how long the wait will be and give an explanation for any delay, if possible. This may help avoid tempers becoming frayed. It is also useful to have a League of Friends snack bar to be able to direct patients and relatives to, where they can while away the time and prevent hypoglycaemia setting in, literally in the case of diabetics.

All patients visiting the outpatient department have their visual acuity recorded, this usually being the responsibility of the nurse. Other nursing procedures (see Chapter 3) may include:

- lacrimal sac washouts;
- epilation of lashes;
- taking conjunctival swabs;
- removing sutures;
- removing/inserting contact lenses;
- instilling drops/ointment;
- removing/inserting prostheses;
- testing for dry eyes using tear strips;
- applying pad and bandaging;
- recording blood pressure, as hypertension can be associated with retinopathies and central artery and vein occlusions. The blood pressure will need to be recorded if the patient is to undergo surgery and for general screening;
- testing urine and/or BM Stix to ensure the patient is not diabetic, as

diabetes can cause various ophthalmic conditions (see Section 16.1), and for general screening.

Minor surgery and investigations will be carried out in the outpatient department. The nurse will need to become familiar with the procedures and instruments and may perform the investigations herself. The operations are performed under local anaesthetic:

- incision and curettage of chalazion;
- lid surgery;
- removal of lid tumours;
- retropunctal cautery;
- 3-snip operation;
- tonometry;
- perimetry;
- biometry.

The UKCC *Scope of Professional Practice* (UKCC 1992) has led to nurses in outpatient departments expanding their practice to encompass nurse-led clinics in areas such as glaucoma and diabetic screening and cataracts.

The optometrist and prosthetist also have clinics in this department.

The high number of patients attending the outpatient department poses particular problems for the nurse, as she will be unable to learn of each one's individual needs. She must be aware of those patients who require particular attention in respect of their communication and mobility difficulties. These difficulties may result from visual impairment or other physical impairments or both. These patients will usually be elderly although not always.

The nurse is unable to see every patient as he leaves the department to ensure that he has understood any prescribed treatment or follow-up. However, she must look out for the elderly and hard of hearing in particular in order to explain any necessary information that the doctor may have given. This information should be supported by written leaflets.

Some patients will have received bad news from the doctor. Those with senile macular degeneration, for example, will have hoped for treatment to improve their eyesight, only to be told that there is little that can be done apart from providing aids to assist with poor vision. The nurse should be aware of these patients and be available to talk to them, answer their questions and refer them to a social worker if appropriate.

The ophthalmic trained nurse will be able to give information to the patient who is to be booked to come into hospital for an operation. She will be able to inform the patient of the approximate length of the waiting time for the operation, what it entails, and the length of the hospital stay. She will be able to answer any queries the patient may have. Some centres are attempting to commence patient assessment in the outpatient department in order that any problems can be anticipated. This is not always feasible when the waiting list entails a delay of more than a few months, as the patient's circumstances may alter in the intervening time. However, the idea itself is sound.

It is of benefit to the patient if he can be shown the ward or day case area. This helps allay fears of coming into hospital and is especially helpful to children and their parents.

The ophthalmic nurse working in the outpatient department has to deal with many patients in the course of a day. She needs to have sound ophthalmic knowledge to be able to attend to the wide variety of ophthalmic conditions with which the patients present in order to give advice and to perform procedures knowledgeably. She needs to be competent in carrying out these nursing procedures and to be aware of the special needs of the elderly, the very young, the deaf, the infirm and the anxious in particular.

## 2.6   THE NURSE IN THE CASUALTY DEPARTMENT

The ophthalmic nurse working in the casualty department is in a similar environment and requires the same sort of skills as the nurse working in the outpatient department. Many people are seen in the casualty area and some of the nursing procedures are the same. In addition, the nurse must be able to deal with emergencies and decide on priority of care. The following conditions are considered ophthalmic emergencies and the patients will require immediate attention:

- sudden loss of vision due to:
  (a)   central retinal artery occlusion (see Section 12.6.2);
  (b)   central retinal vein occlusion (see Section 12.6.3);
  (c)   giant cell arteritis (see Section 16.5);
  (d)   retinal detachment – especially if the macula is still attached (see Section 12.6.1);
- primary acute glaucoma (see Section 10.7.1);
- trauma, especially penetrating or perforating injuries (see Section 14.1);
- chemical burns (see Section 14.7);
- orbital cellulitis (see Section 5.3.1).

Urgent cases the nurse may have to deal with which are not classed as emergencies include:

- corneal ulcer (see Section 8.5.2);
- vitreous haemorrhage (see Section 12.9.3);
- acute dacryocystitis (see Section 6.5.2);

- optic nerve disorders (see Section 12.8);
- ocular tumours (see Section 9.5.3);
- acute uveitis (see Section 9.5.2).

The nurse will need to inform the waiting patients of the approximate waiting time and she may need to explain that some people require priority care and will be attended to as soon as they arrive in the department.

It is the nurse's responsibility to take a good history and decide what priority, if any, the patient should be given. She must give details of the state of the patient's vision on arrival and of the type of injury or eye complaint. The importance of taking an accurate history cannot be over emphasised. The history may give clues to the type of injury sustained that is not evident on initial eye examination. The history must include the following items.

- *Visual acuity.* This can be used for medico-legal purposes especially if an accident has occurred at work and damages might be claimed.
- *Type of injury.*
    - (a)  If a foreign body entered the eye:
        - (i)    what the foreign body was;
        - (ii)   when the accident happened;
        - (iii)  how it got into the eye. It is especially important to find out whether the patient was using a hammer and chisel, and if the foreign body hit the eye with force, which might indicate that it had penetrated the eye, in which case an orbital X-ray would need to be ordered;
        - (iv)  if protective goggles were being worn at the time of the incident.
    - (b)  If a fluid substance has entered the eye:
        - (i)    what the substance is;
        - (ii)   when the incident occurred;
        - (iii)  whether it was washed out immediately.
    - (c)  If the eye has been scratched:
        - (i)    what scratched the eye;
        - (ii)   with what force it did so;
        - (iii)  when the incident occurred.
- *Type of eye complaint.* The nurse must elicit whether the following symptoms are present and their duration:
    - (a)  discharge, especially on waking;
    - (b)  watering;
    - (c)  photophobia;
    - (d)  pain or discomfort, its location and nature;
    - (e)  change in vision:
        - (i)    blurred vision;
        - (ii)   floaters;

(iii)   visual loss – sudden
                       gradual
                       total
                       partial – which visual field is affected.

If the patient has had an accident, he may need to be treated for shock. Any accompanying relatives or friends may also be shocked and anxious.

Patients suffering from sudden loss of vision will be anxious, as will those who are to be admitted to hospital, especially if this is unexpected. The nurse must help alleviate these fears and anxieties. She can offer practical help such as informing relatives or arranging transport.

The nurse will be expected to carry out varied nursing procedures in the casualty department (see Chapter 3):

- the taking and recording of visual acuity;
- examination of the eye – this may be carried out using a torch or with a slit lamp;
- instillation of drops and ointment;
- removal of conjunctival and superficial corneal foreign bodies;
- application of pad and bandaging;
- irrigation of the eye;
- epilation of lashes;
- syringing of the lacrimal ducts;
- removal of sutures;
- removal/insertion of contact lenses;
- removal/insertion of prostheses;
- testing urine;
- recording BM Stix;
- recording blood pressure;
- taking conjunctival swabs;
- performing tear strip test for dry eyes.

The nurse must remember while performing these procedures that the patient may feel faint or unwell.

The nurse in the casualty department must be able to deal with many people and to cope with unexpected situations which might arise. She must have adequate ophthalmic knowledge to be able to recognise urgent cases and to be able to give certain patients priority care. She also needs to be able to perform a variety of ophthalmic procedures competently and knowledgeably.

This is an ideal time to carry out patient education by giving out relevant information leaflets and informing patients on eye protection as appropriate. The nurse in casualty also advises patients over the telephone so it is vital that her knowledge is accurate and her communication skills are appropriate.

## 2.7    THE DAY CASE AND WARD NURSE

Most of the patients in the ophthalmic ward will require pre- and post-operative care, as the majority are admitted for surgery, e.g. cataract extraction; squint surgery; repair of retinal detachment; drainage surgery for chronic glaucoma; following trauma. There may, however, be patients admitted for rest following trauma or vitreous haemorrhage, for intensive treatment of a severe infection, or for treatment of herpes zoster ophthalmics.

The specific nursing care for each ophthalmic condition is detailed in the relevant chapters. However, a general note on nursing care is given here.

### 2.7.1    Pre-assessment

Patients having day case or inpatient surgery tend to be pre-assessed a few weeks prior to the operation. This is carried out to assess the needs of the individual patient in order to be able to plan their short period in hospital, to give the necessary information regarding the surgery and to plan with the patient and carers their care following the operation.

The care following surgery will involve instillation of drops which in the majority of cases will be performed by the patient himself or his carer. Ideally teaching on drop instillation should be instituted at pre-assessment as there is little time for this during the admission to hospital. Advising patients to purchase artificial tear drops and practice at home following instruction is one way of overcoming the lack of time there is to carry out this teaching and observation of the patient's performance.

The nurse has only limited time in which to assess the needs of the patients and must apply all her assessment skills appropriately (see Section 2.3).

As well as giving the usual pre-operative information to the patient, the nurse may carry out the following procedures:

- visual acuity (see Section 3.2.2);
- tonometry (see Section 3.2.25);
- biometry (see Section 3.2.27);
- ECG;
- focimetry.

Information leaflets regarding the surgery (see Patient Information Leaflet No. 2) and hospital stay should be given to the patient to support the verbal information and instructions that the nurse will give. These can be translated into languages other than English if necessary. This, together with answering any queries the patient or carer may have, will help allay fears.

## PATIENT INFORMATION LEAFLET No. 2

# DAY CASE CATARACT SURGERY

This leaflet outlines information relating to day case cataract surgery. It will introduce you to what you need to know before your operation, what to expect on the day, and some guidelines for when you return home.

Day case cataract surgery enables you to come into hospital in the morning or afternoon and return to your own home on the same day.

At the Eye Unit we have a purpose built department for day case. Our aim is to provide a comfortable and friendly atmosphere during your short stay with us. The Day Case Team have certain criteria to fulfil. To enable us to achieve this we will send you a questionnaire. This refers to the care you may have available at home.

You will be asked:

- If you have transport to and from the Eye Unit on the day of your operation and the day after.
- If you have a companion to come with you.
- If someone is able to stay with you or are you able to stay with someone the night after your operation.
- If you have access to a telephone.
- If you are willing to have a local anaesthetic.

### Before your surgery

Approximately two to four weeks before your operation you will be sent an appointment to attend a pre-assessment clinic. At this clinic you will receive information and advice concerning your operation. This will include written and verbal instruction about what will happen to you before, during and after your operation. You will also have an appointment to see a doctor, who will assess any medical problems.

The nursing staff are available to answer any questions you may have, and there will be an opportunity for you to visit the day case unit. At this visit you will also be given the date of your operation.

### On the day of your operation

You should arrive promptly at the appointed time with your companion, who should be a friend or relative, at the Eye Unit reception.

One of the Day Case Team will escort you and your companion to the day case unit.

Ensure that you bring:

- All your current medication (including tablets, eye drops, etc.) labelled in their own original containers.
- A dressing gown if you have one, a pair of indoor shoes, cotton brief clean pair of socks.

## PATIENT INFORMATION LEAFLET No. 2 *continued*

We advise you to wear loose, comfortable clothing so as to avoid pulling tight garments over your head after surgery.

We ask ladies not to wear make-up, nail varnish or excess jewellery.

We advise you not to bring any items of value. Please leave them at home. There are no storage facilities for such articles at the hospital.

After your operation, you will be offered light refreshments.

Because of the advances in local anaesthetics and the technique of up-to-date cataract surgery you and your companion will be able to return home relatively soon after the operation. Written and verbal information will be given before you depart.

We will advise your companion when you will be ready to leave. They are very welcome to stay with you before and after your operation or visit the various shops and cafes at the hospital.

### After your operation

For the remainder of the day we advise you to rest and avoid any heavy lifting or straining.

The next day you will be required to return to the Eye Unit for the first dressing. At this point the day case nurse will remove the dressing, bathe the eye and instil eye drops. You will then be seen by the doctor. If all is well you and your companion will be given advice and information to ensure continued healing.

The Day Case Cataract Team hope that this leaflet will give you an outline of the care you will receive as a day case patient.

If you require any further information please contact the Day Case Team on ...........

### How to get there

By bus:


By Car:


...... .......

## 2.7.2   Pre-operative care

In addition to the routine pre-operative care for surgery being performed under either local or general anaesthesia, the nurse may be required to carry out the following procedures, depending on the personal preferences of the ophthalmic surgeon (see Chapter 3):

- taking conjunctival swabs for culture and sensitivity tests;
- lacrimal syringing;
- instilling antibiotic drops, e.g. G. chloramphenicol either 4 times a day for 1 or 2 days, or intensively, for example, every 15 minutes for 2 hours immediately prior to surgery to prevent post-operative infection;
- instilling mydriatic drops prior to cataract extraction or retinal detachment surgery as the pupil needs to be dilated for such surgery to be performed. These drops are usually administered intensively, e.g. every 15 minutes for 1–2 hours before surgery;
- instilling miotic drops prior to trabeculectomy and keratoplasty;
- instilling local anaesthetic drops if the operation is to be performed under a local anaesthetic. Drops such as G. cocaine hydrochloride 2–5% or G. amethocaine hydrochloride 0.5–1% are instilled every 5–15 minutes for up to an hour before surgery. A cartella shield must be put over the eye to protect it once it is anaesthetised.

## 2.7.3   Post-operative care

In addition to the normal post-operative care required by any patient after surgery, the nurse will need to follow a routine such as that described here, although this will vary to some extent according to hospital practice.

- Eye care:
  (a) dressings – the eye will usually only be cleaned once before discharge or on the day following day case surgery, unless the patient is kept in hospital longer. Cleaning may then be performed twice a day;
  (b) inspection of the eye – the eye will be examined post-operatively (see Chapter 3, Nursing Procedures);
  (c) instillation of drops – antibiotic drops may be instilled hourly, two hourly, or four times a day; a steroid and mydriatic drop may be used; ointment may be applied at night;
  (d) protection of the eye – eye pads or cartella shields may be worn on the first post-operative day. Cartella shields are usually worn at night for two weeks.
- Discharge: All patients should be given instructions about care and follow-up:

(a) eyedrops – patient's and carer's ability to instil drops should be checked. Ideally this will have commenced at pre-assessment. Names of drops and times of instillation must be written down. A cartella shield should be given for night wear;

(b) cleaning the eye – if the eye is sticky in the mornings, it should be cleaned using cooled, boiled water and cotton wool or gauze. Advise patients never to use dry cotton wool near the eye, as fibres can get into it;

(c) general instructions – the patients must not stoop down too low in case they lose their balance or do anything causing increased exertion that will raise the intra-ocular pressure, such as lifting anything heavy. Patients should have their hair washed while bending backwards over the basin. All these restrictions should be heeded for two weeks initially but are becoming increasingly less necessary with small incision surgery. They must especially take care not to knock the eye, which could cause haemorrhage or the iris to prolapse through the wound;

(d) outpatient appointment – ensure that the patient has an appointment, usually for one or two weeks following discharge. Transport may need to be arranged for the day;

(e) primary care – the nurse may need to arrange for a district nurse, home help, meals on wheels, for the patient prior to discharge;

(f) convalescence – in some areas recuperation in a convalescent or nursing home can be arranged for patients before they return to their own homes.

It is helpful if all the above information and instructions are written down as well as given verbally, as there is often much detail to absorb in the excitement of going home.

### 2.7.4  Nursing procedures

The ophthalmic nurse working on the ward and in day case needs to be able to assess the patients and plan their care on an individual basis. She must understand the pre- and post-operative care required for each type of ophthalmic operation. She needs to be able to carry out certain ophthalmic procedures competently and knowledgeably. The nurse must also plan the patient's discharge, in advance, ensuring that all relevant agencies are involved. She must be knowledgeable in all ophthalmic aspects in order to discuss relevant points with the patient and relatives so that the hospital stay can be made as easy and pleasant as possible for all concerned.

## 2.8 THE NURSE IN THE THEATRE

The nurse working in an ophthalmic theatre will need to be familiar with the nursing responsibilities and general duties required of any theatre nurse. In addition she will need to know the following aspects of ophthalmic theatre nursing, though the details will vary from hospital to hospital.

### 2.8.1 Preparation of the patient

Once on the operating table, the patient must be positioned correctly, especially if a general anaesthetic is being administered. A Rubens pillow is used to position and support the adult patient's head and a head ring for a child. Local anaesthetic drops, if no general anaesthetic is to be given, may be instilled prior to the operation commencing.

If the patient is having the operation under a local anaesthetic, it is important that a nurse sits and holds his hand during the procedure. This not only reassures the patient but can give the nurse an indication of his condition. Intravenous sedatives, e.g. diazepam, may be given to the patient.

During the operation the patient's face will be covered with a sterile towel. This may make the patient feel claustrophobic and perhaps disorientated. Usually a supply of oxygen at 4 litres per minute with an air intake or air alone is administered to the patient. If oxygen is being given, the supply must be switched off if cautery is used as it constitutes a fire hazard.

The nurse holding the patient's hand will be able to take the pulse, observe the colour of the finger nails and watch the chest movements. She will also feel any pressure from the patient's hand indicating that he may be feeling discomfort or pain.

### 2.8.2 Knowledge of the instruments

The nurse must have a good knowledge of the instruments required for each operation performed on the eye. The suture materials used in ophthalmic surgery tend to be very fine, 10/0 nylon, 10/0 prolene or 8/0 virgin silk for intra-ocular surgery often being used.

### 2.8.3 Technique in handling the instruments

Preferably a non-touch technique is carried out, using forceps to handle the needles and sutures. The tips of the instruments should not be touched with the fingers.

### 2.8.4   The wearing of gloves

Gloves with powder must not be used as the starch it contains is an irritant to the eye. Surgical gloves containing no powder are available such as Biogel M worn by surgeons and scrub nurses for microsurgery.

### 2.8.5   Care of the instruments

Ophthalmic instruments tend to be small, delicate and expensive, and great care must be taken when handling them. They must be cleaned carefully and thoroughly using a toothbrush, general purpose cleanser or ultrasonic bath.

Each instrument must be seen to be in good working order, not rusted or damaged, and should be checked under a magnified light source before being sterilised. Sharp instruments should be sterilised in a tray or rack with their ends protected by silicone tubing. Most instruments are sterilised in hot air ovens, usually at a temperature of 160°C for 1 hour. Browne's control tubes, a chemical indicator and hot air tape are used to indicate that the machine has attained a specified temperature but the oven should be checked annually or biannually to ensure that complete sterilisation is taking place. Instruments can also be sterilised commercially using ethylene oxide and gamma irradiation. Autoclaves, steam under pressure, are used for tubing and any other plastic items, e.g. microscope caps, that cannot withstand the 160°C of the hot air ovens.

### 2.8.6   The operation and use of equipment

The nurse must be familiar with the equipment used in the ophthalmic theatre:

- the operating microscope which is used for most intra-ocular surgery;
- the cryotherapy machine used for retinal detachment surgery;
- Phako emulsifier machines which are used for extracapsular cataract extractions and for vitrectomy surgery;
- magnets used for removing intra-ocular and intracorneal magnetic foreign bodies. Magnetic instruments are used with the magnet and must be demagnetised following use;
- cautery machines:
  - (a)  bipolar cautery is used on the eye and no diathermy plate is required;
  - (b)  macropolar cautery is used on lids and does require a diathermy plate;
- laser operating loops.

The nurse working in the ophthalmic theatre must appreciate the delicate nature of the surgery taking place. She needs to understand the importance of quietness, speed, attentiveness, cleanliness and sterility. The nurse must also know the particular procedures for each ophthalmic operation at which she will be assisting and be prepared to develop her knowledge as new procedures and instruments are introduced.

# 3 Ophthalmic Nursing Procedures

## 3.1 GENERAL PRINCIPLES

Ophthalmic nursing procedures will vary to some degree between hospitals or units. Those listed here can be used as guidelines but local policies must be followed.

Certain general principles should be followed in all ophthalmic procedures.

- Explain to the patient what you are going to do.
- Ensure that the patient is sitting or lying with his head well supported.
- Ensure that there is a good light source.
- Wear your prescribed glasses for near vision if applicable, or use a loupe or magnifying glasses such as Bishop Harmann's spectacles, if necessary.
- Always wash your hands at the start and completion of each procedure and during the procedure as necessary, e.g. after removing a soiled dressing and before touching the eye again.
- Ask the patient to move the eye being examined so that the cornea is moved away from the area you are dealing with. This is particularly important in order to prevent accidental corneal damage if the eye is anaesthetised.
- Be gentle and dexterous.
- Support your hands against the patient's face so that if he suddenly moves, your hands will move as well, preventing instruments touching the eye.

## 3.2 NURSING PROCEDURES

### 3.2.1 Instilling drops and ointment

**Equipment**

Assemble relevant drops and/or ointment, prescription sheet, box of tissues/gauze swabs.

| Procedure | Rationale |
| --- | --- |
| **1** Check identity of the patient and drops/ointment with assistant if available. | To ensure the correct patient receives the correct drops/ointment and to obtain the patient's consent and co-operation. |
| **2** Position hand holding bottle/dropper/tube gently on patient's forehead. | To prevent bottle/dropper/tube touching patient's eye if moved. |
| **3** Hold down lower lid with tissue/gauze square in other hand. | To expose conjunctival sac into which drop/ointment can be instilled. |
| **4** Ask the patient to look up. | So that drop falls into lower fornix and not onto the cornea which would cause patient to blink. |
| **5** Instil one drop into lower fornix towards outer canthus **or** squeeze 5 mm ointment along lower fornix from inner canthus towards outer canthus. | If drop is instilled near inner canthus it will drain straight down the tear duct before it is of any therapeutic value. Only one drop to be instilled at one time as additional drops will overflow. |
| **6** Release lid and ask patient to gently close eye for a few moments without squeezing. | To allow time for absorption of drops. |
| **7** Gently wipe away excess drops or ointment. | For patient's comfort and to prevent possible drug irritation on skin. |
| **8** Dispose of tissue/gauze squares in nearest clinical waste bin. | |
| **9** Sign prescription sheet. | To indicate drops have been administered. |

### 3.2.2 Recording visual acuity

This procedure records the acuteness of central vision for distance, and near or reading vision.

**Distance vision** (Fig. 3.1)

Distance vision is tested at 6 m as rays of light from this distance are nearly parallel. If the patient wears glasses constantly, vision may be recorded with and without glasses, but this must be noted on the record. Each eye is tested and recorded separately, the other being covered with a card held by the examiner.

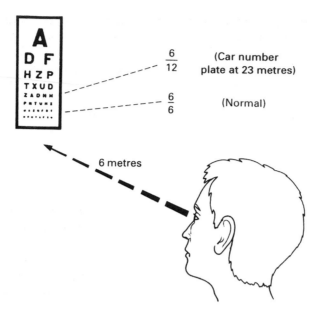

**Fig. 3.1** Testing distance visual acuity.

*Snellen's test type*

Heavy block letters, numbers or symbols printed in black on a white background, are arranged on a chart in 9 rows of graded size, diminishing from above downwards. The top letter can be read by the normal eye at a distance of 60 m, and the following rows should be read at 36, 24, 18, 12, 9, 6, 5, 4 m respectively.

The patient is seated 6 m from the chart, which must be adequately lit, and asked to read down to the smallest letter he can distinguish, using one eye at a time.

*Visual acuity* is expressed as a fraction and abbreviated as VA. The *numerator* is the distance in metres at which a person can read a given line of letters. The *denominator* is the distance at which a person with normal average vision can read the same line, e.g. if the 7th line is read at a distance of 6 m this is VA 6/6. If some letters in the line are read but not all, it is expressed as, for example, VA 6/6 −2, or VA 6/9 +2.

For vision less than 6/60 the distance between the patient and the chart is reduced a metre at a time and the vision is recorded accordingly as, for example, 5/60, 4/60, 3/60, 2/60, 1/60.

If the patient cannot read the top letter at a distance of 1 metre, the examiner's hand is held at 0.9 m, 0.6 m or 0.3 m away against a dark background and the patient is asked to count the number of fingers held up. If he answers correctly, record VA = CF (count fingers). For less vision the hand is moved in front of the eye at 0.3 m, record VA = HM (hand movement).

In the case of less vision, test for projection of light by shining a torch into the eye from different directions to see if the patient can tell from which direction it comes. If he sees the light but not the direction, it is noted as VA = PL (perception of light). This test is performed in a dark room. If no light is seen, record NO PL, which is total blindness. A 'pinhole disc' is used if the VA is less than 6/6 or 6/9, which may improve VA. If considerable increase in vision is obtained, it may usually be assumed that there is no gross abnormality, but a refractive error.

### Near vision

Near vision is tested by cards consisting of different sizes of ordinary printer's type; each size being numbered. The eyes are tested and recorded separately, and if the patient uses reading glasses, these should be worn during the test.

The card is held at a comfortable distance (approximately 25 cm) and should be well illuminated by a light from behind the patient's shoulder. The near vision is recorded as the card number of the smallest size type he can most easily read.

### 3.2.3   Dressing the eye

### Equipment

Trolley with eye dressing pack, plus:

- sterile normal saline
- steret
- scissors
- pen torch
- pad
- tape
- extra gauze squares
- bag for rubbish

| Procedure | Rationale |
|---|---|
| 1  Prepare trolley according to local policies. | |
| 2  Identify the patient. | To ensure the correct patient receives treatment and to obtain the patient's consent and co-operation. |
| 3  Open the pack and prepare the sterile surface. | So areas of potential contamination are kept to a minimum. |
| 4  Remove eye pad from patient if present. | |

▶

5   Clean the eye with eyes closed. Use one swab only, cleaning from the inside outwards.

6   Clean along lower eyelid margin, asking the patient to look up and everting the lower lid. Use one swab only, cleaning from the inside outwards.

To ensure the eye is clean with no risk of contamination and to protect other ocular structures.

7   Clean along the upper lid margin by asking the patient to look down as you gently elevate the lid away from the globe. Use one swab only, cleaning from the inside outwards.

8   Repeat if necessary. If there is stubborn discharge, lay a wet swab over the eye for a few minutes to loosen it.

9   Inspect the eye using a torch.

To observe for any abnormalities.

10   Instil prescribed drops/ointment or observe patient/carer doing so.

To ensure patient receives correct medication appropriately.

### 3.2.4   Applying pad and bandage

#### Pads

Pads are usually applied to patients with corneal abrasions. However, Kirkpatrick *et al.* (1993) found that the corneal epithelium healing rate was significantly improved without a pad. Patients with large abrasions may find a pad and perhaps a bandage affords more comfort if applied firmly as the eyelid is prevented from irritating the abrasion.

If a pad is to be applied, it is important that the eye is firmly closed under the pad to avoid corneal abrasion. In some instances it is useful to apply a piece of paraffin gauze over the eyelids, then a pad or half a pad folded in two and finally a pad applied flat over the eye. This method is useful in the casualty or outpatient departments but should not be used on post-operative patients as it will put too much pressure on the globe, unless pressure needs to be applied post-operatively, e.g. to seal a leaking wound. Secure the pad with three pieces of tape. For the right eye, the first piece of tape should be placed over the centre of the pad, diagonally from 1 to 7 o'clock. For the left eye, it is placed diagonally from 11 to 5 o'clock. The second and third pieces of tape are placed each side of this central piece, parallel to it. Position the ends of each piece of tape on each other so that removal is easier and kinder to the patient.

*Disadvantages of eye pads*

- Corneal abrasion can be caused if the eye is not closed under the pad.
- Good medium for bacterial growth.
- They are flammable.
- Uncomfortable to wear.
- If the lids are swollen, a lid abrasion may occur.
- Corneal healing rate reduced (Kirkpatrick *et al.* 1993).

## Bandages

There are several different methods of applying an eye bandage. One method is described here which provides a secure, comfortable, effective result.

(1)  Take the bandage once around the forehead.
(2)  Bring it up under the ear on the affected side and over the centre of the eye pad.
(3)  Repeat this twice more, covering the eye pad above and below the first central turn.
(4)  Take the bandage once more around the forehead and secure it.

### 3.2.5   Inspecting the eye

#### Casualty

When examining a patient's eye, first look at the patient's face as a whole to ensure facial symmetry and note any obvious palsy, ptosis, proptosis, or allergic reaction. The eye is always examined from the outside inwards. If only one eye is affected, inspect the 'good' eye first for comparison.

Ask the patient to open both eyes as this is easier than to open one eye alone. Use a good pen torch or slit lamp. Ensure that the patient's head is well supported. If the patient is in pain, local anaesthetic drops may be necessary. If there is a history of glass or fibreglass in the eye or the history indicates possible penetrating injury or perforation, local anaesthetic should not be instilled. The reason for the former is to more easily identify if the glass/fibreglass has been removed, the latter to avoid the drug entering the eye.

Always consider the patient's age and psychological state.

*Eyelids.* Look for:
- ptosis
- swelling
- discoloration
- discharge/crusting

- ingrowing lashes
- entropion
- ectropion
- laceration

*Conjunctiva.* Look for:
- injection (redness)
- degree of injection
- position of injection
  (a) limbal/ciliary
  (b) localised – with or without dilated episcleral vessels
  (c) generalised
- subconjunctival haemorrhage
- chemosis (swelling)
- foreign body
- laceration
- cysts
- pinguecula
- pterygium
- follicles
- papillae

*Cornea.* Look for:
- clarity
- foreign body
- abrasion
- laceration
- ulcers

*Anterior chamber.* Assess:
- depth (should be deep but compare with other eye)
Look for:
- hyphaema
- hypopyon
- flare and cells (using slit lamp)

*Iris.* Assess:
- colour – compare with other eye
- clarity and pattern
Look for:
- iridodialysis

*Pupil.* Assess:
- shape (should be round – an irregular pupil could indicate synaechiae, an oval pupil could indicate acute glaucoma)

- size
- reaction
- position (should be central)
- colour – usually black. The red reflex may be noted. (A white or grey pupil suggests the presence of a cataract. A white pupil in a baby/child indicates a cataract or retinoblastoma.)

**Post-operatively**

The eye is examined from outside inwards. The eye pad (if worn) is inspected for discharge/blood.

*Eyelids.* Look for:
- swelling
- discoloration
- discharge/crusting
- entropion (from bad padding technique)
- bruising from local anaesthetic injection

*Conjunctiva.* Look for:
- injection (redness)
- subconjunctival haemorrhage
- chemosis (oedema)
- section – intact suture line – iris prolapse
- presence of bleb post-trabeculectomy
- presence of entry sites post-vitrectomy

*Cornea.* Look for:
- clarity
- abrasion

*Anterior chamber.* Assess:
- depth (should be deep but compare with other eye)

Look for:
- hyphaema
- hypopyon

*Iris.* Look for:
- peripheral iridectomy/iridotomy (may be too small to see)

*Pupil.* Assess:
- shape (a peaked pupil may indicate an iris prolapse)
- size (may be dilated with mydriatics; may be miosed with miotics)
- reaction (will not react if mydriatics or miotics are being instilled)

- position
- colour – should be black. The red reflex may be noted.

### 3.2.6   Taking a conjunctival swab

#### Equipment

- Correct culture medium and swab stick. Different ones are required for bacteria, viruses and *Chlamydia.*
- Appropriate pathology form.

| Procedure | Rationale |
|---|---|
| 1  Identify patient and check what type of swab is required. | To ensure the correct patient receives the correct procedure and to obtain the patient's consent and co-operation. |
| 2  Wash hands. | To prevent infection from transient organisms. |
| 3  Assemble equipment. If both eyes are to be swabbed label swabs 'right' and 'left'. | To prevent wrong swab being placed in medium. |
| 4  Ask the patient to look up. | To prevent corneal damage. |
| 5  Swab firmly along lower fornix from nasal side outwards. When taking swab for *Chlamydia* more pressure is needed to obtain the organisms from the follicles. *Note:* Swabs should be taken before G. fluorescein, or a topical anaesthetic, has been instilled. | To sweep organisms away from lower punctum. To obtain as many organisms as possible. |
| 6  Place stick in culture bottle. | |
| 7  Wash hands. | To prevent cross infection. |
| 8  Label bottle and send to laboratory. | For process to continue. |

### 3.2.7   Performing epilation of eyelashes

Ingrowing eyelashes (*trichiasis*) may be removed by epilation to give temporary relief from symptoms caused by their constant irritation of the cornea and conjunctiva.

## Equipment

- Epilation forceps
- Tissues
- Fluorescein minims
- Good light or slit lamp

| Procedure | Rationale |
|---|---|
| **1** Identify the patient. | To ensure the correct patient receives treatment and to obtain the patient's consent and co-operation. |
| **2** Sit patient with head supported. | To ensure safety and patient comfort. |
| **3** Evert lid slightly – for lower lid ask the patient to look up; for upper lid ask the patient to look down. | To prevent ocular damage and for ease of performance. |
| **4** Remove the lash by gripping it at its root with the epilation forceps and pulling firmly in the direction of the hair growth. | For ease of performance and to minimise discomfort for patient. To ensure hair root is removed. |
| **5** Instil with fluorescein. | To see if the cornea is staining. If this occurs, a prophylactic antibiotic, e.g. Chloromycetin, may be prescribed. |

The treatment must be repeated as often as required by the patient, e.g. weekly, monthly, as necessary.

Patients or carers with good vision may be able to perform epilation themselves at home.

## Electrolysis

Electrolysis is used to remove ingrowing lashes by means of a needle electrode applied to the lash follicle. It is a painful procedure and the lid is first anaesthetised with a local anaesthetic injection.

## Cryotherapy

Cryotherapy can be used to remove lashes by applying liquid nitrogen to the offending lash follicle. This is performed by the doctor but the nurse needs to prepare the patient.

### Equipment

- Local anaesthetic drops, e.g. proxymetacaine hydrochloride 0.5% (Ophthaine)

- Local anaesthetic injection, e.g. lignocaine hydrochloride 2%
- 2 ml syringe
- Green and orange needles
- Paraffin gauze
- 'Shoe horn'
- Lubricant (K-Y) jelly
- Sterile cotton wool buds
- Dressing towel
- Tissues
- Epilation forceps
- Liquid nitrogen (cryo) container

| Procedure | Rationale |
| --- | --- |
| 1 Identify the patient. | To ensure the correct patient receives treatment and to obtain the patient's consent and co-operation. |
| 2 Lie the patient on the bed. | For patient comfort and to aid procedure. |
| 3 Instil prescribed local anaesthetic drops. | To reduce discomfort. |
| 4 Prepare local anaesthetic injection. | To reduce discomfort. |
| 5 Insert 'shoe horn', well lubricated with jelly, into appropriate fornix. | To protect anterior surface of eye. |
| 6 Cover the patient's head with dressing towel. | To protect area around lid being treated. |
| 7 Fill cryo container with liquid nitrogen. | To assist with procedure. |
| 8 Put cotton wool buds into liquid nitrogen and pass to doctor when ready. | To assist with procedure. |
| 9 Pass epilation forceps when required by the doctor. | To assist with procedure. |

The patient should be warned that lid(s) may become inflamed.

Cryotherapy is not used on patients with symblepharon.

### 3.2.8   Everting the upper lid

The upper lid is everted to inspect the palpebral conjunctiva over the subtarsal area. Foreign bodies or conjunctival follicles may be present.

## Equipment

- Glass rod
- Good light or slit lamp

| Procedure | Rationale |
|---|---|
| **(A) Chair method** | |
| **1** Tell the patient what you are going to do. Warn the patient that there will be a peculiar sensation. | To obtain the patient's consent and co-operation. |
| **2** Stand behind the patient, supporting the patient's head against your body. | For support and ease of performance. |
| **3** Ask the patient to look downwards. | To enable lid to be everted. |
| **4** Take hold of the lashes of the upper lid with one hand and gently pull forwards and downwards. | To enable lid to be everted. |
| **5** With the other hand, use a glass rod or finger and place over tarsal plate (mid lid area). | To enable lid to be everted. |
| **6** Push gently into the tarsal plate, at the same time the hand holding the lashes everts the lid. | To enable lid to be everted. |
| **7** Tell the patient to keep looking down. | To maintain eversion. |
| **8** Inspect the sub-tarsal conjunctiva. | To examine for abnormalities. |
| **(B) Slit lamp method** | |
| Use the above method but approach the patient from the front. | |
| **To reposition the lid** | |
| Ask the patient to look up and blink. | To reposition upper lid. |

## 3.2.9 Removing a foreign body from the conjunctiva or cornea

## Equipment

- Sterile cotton wool buds
- Sterile water
- Local anaesthetic drops

| Procedure | Rationale |
|---|---|
| **1** Identify the patient. Sit the patient comfortably with head well supported. | To obtain the patient's consent and co-operation and for safety. |
| **2** Instil local anaesthetic drops (*not* usually necessary for a sub-tarsal foreign body). | To reduce discomfort. |
| **3** Using a wet cotton wool bud swab, gently wipe away the foreign body. | To ensure no dry fibres enter the eye. |
| **4** Instil G. fluorescein. | To see if abrasion resulted and treat if necessary. |

### 3.2.10    Taping the lower lid to relieve entropion

As a temporary measure the lower lid can be taped to relieve an entropion. A piece of micropore tape about 1.3 to 2.5 cm ($\frac{1}{4}$ to 1 inch) in length is applied just below the lower lid margin and secured on the cheek in such a way as to bring the lower lid into its normal position.

### 3.2.11    Testing for dry eyes using tear strips

This test is performed to discern if the eyes are dry (see Section 6.5.4). It is a test of the quantity not quality of the tear film (Ragge & Easty 1990).

### Equipment

- Tear test strips
- Timer or watch
- Local anaesthetic

| Procedure | Rationale |
|---|---|
| **1** Identify the patient. | To ensure the correct patient receives the test and is prepared. |
| **2** Instil local anaesthetic drops if prescribed. | To anaesthetise the eye for patient comfort. |
| **3** Prepare strips in accordance with instructions on the packet. | To ensure the test is carried out correctly. |
| **4** Ask the patient to look up and insert the strip in accordance with the manufacturer's instructions. | To ensure the test is carried out correctly. |
| It is helpful to mark the strip R and L as appropriate. | To avoid confusion between eyes. |

▶

| 5 | The patient may open or close his eyes during the procedure. | To ensure patient comfort. |

| 6 | After 5 minutes remove the strips and read off the result against the scale on the packet.<br>Record the result in the patient's notes as follows:<br>Right = $n$ mm in 5 mins<br>Left = $n$ mm in 5 mins<br>If the whole strip is wet record the result as +++ | For a permanent record in the patient's notes. |

### 3.2.12   Irrigating the eye

Irrigation of the eye is performed to clean the eye thoroughly of all foreign substances, especially corrosive matter. As an emergency measure, speedy dilution of any substance is very important and irrigating the eye immediately with the nearest tap water may greatly reduce the amount of damage to the tissues.

### Equipment

- Litmus paper
- Bottle of universal buffer solution **or** bottle of sterile water **or** bottle of sodium chloride **or** continuous flow irrigation
- Undine for use with buffer solution
- Local anaesthetic drops
- Desmarres lid retractor if a chemical injury
- Tissues
- Protective plastic bibs or cape
- Paper towels
- Receptacle for paper towels
- Receiver

| Procedure | Rationale |
|---|---|
| 1  Identify the patient. | To ensure the correct patient receives treatment and to obtain the patient's consent and co-operation. |
| 2  Sit the patient in a chair with his head well supported and turned slightly to the affected side. | To prevent irrigation fluid entering the unaffected eye. |
| 3  Test pH of conjunctival sac. | To ascertain whether substance in eye is alkali or acid. |

▶

| | | |
|---|---|---|
| **4** | Instil anaesthetic drops. | To anaesthetise the eye for patient comfort. |
| **5** | If applicable, warm the irrigating fluid. | For patient comfort. |
| **6** | Place a protective bib and paper towels around the patient's neck. | To protect patient's clothing from getting wet. |
| **7** | Place the receiver against the patient's face on the affected side. Ask the patient to hold it if no other help is available. | To collect the irrigating fluid. |
| **8** | Test warmth of fluid on hand. | To ensure the fluid is not too hot. |
| **9** | When the temperature is suitable run a stream of fluid up the cheek towards the eye. | To prepare the patient for fluid entering the eye. |
| **10** | Evert the lower lid, asking the patient to look up and irrigate the lower fornix. | To ensure all anterior surfaces of the eye, especially the fornices, are irrigated. |
| **11** | Evert the upper lid and irrigate the upper fornix. | To ensure all anterior surfaces of the eye, especially the fornices, are irrigated. |
| **12** | Double evert the upper lid using Desmarres lid retractor if necessary. | To ensure that no solidified material such as cement is in the upper fornix. |
| **13** | Complete the irrigation by asking the patient to move his eye from side to side and up and down, holding the lids open. | To ensure all anterior surfaces of the eye, especially the fornices, are irrigated. |
| **14** | Re-test the pH of the conjunctival sac. | To ensure the pH is within normal limits (7.1–8.6) (Saude 1992). |
| **15** | Repeat irrigation until the pH is normal. | |
| **16** | Wipe patient's face dry. | For patient comfort. |

### Notes:

| | |
|---|---|
| ■ Do not hold the spout too close or too far away from the eye; about 2.5 cm is best. | If too close it may touch the eye; if too far away the stream of fluid may be too harsh. |
| ■ Rest the hand holding the bottle or giving set against the patient's head. | For support and to lessen the chance of the spout entering the eye if the patient should move. |
| ■ It may be necessary to instil local anaesthetic drops over the everted upper lid. | For patient comfort. |

### 3.2.13   Syringing the lacrimal ducts

This is performed to determine whether the lacrimal drainage apparatus is blocked or patent.

### Equipment

Tray or trolley with:

- 2 ml syringe
- 1 lacrimal cannula ⎫
- 1 Nettleship dilator ⎬ sterile
- 1 punctum finder ⎭
- ampule normal saline
- local anaesthetic drops, e.g. pyroxymetacaine hydrochloride 0.5% (Ophthaine)
- box of tissues
- bag for soiled tissues
- torch or good light
- patient's notes

| Procedure | Rationale |
| --- | --- |
| **1** Identify the patient. | To ensure the correct patient receives treatment and to obtain the patient's consent and co-operation. |
| **2** Lie or sit the patient comfortably with head supported. | For patient comfort and safety. |
| **3** Instil local anaesthetic drops over the inner canthus. | To prevent patient discomfort. |
| **4** Fill syringe with saline, attach cannula securely and ensure patency. | For safety and to ensure equipment is not faulty. |
| **5** Stand behind or beside the patient. | To ease performance. |
| **6** Ask the patient to look upwards/ outwards. | To prevent ocular damage. |
| **7** With the right hand, insert the Nettleship dilator into the punctum vertically 1–2 mm. Then gently turn it horizontally towards the nose and carefully rotate it a few times between the finger and thumb to dilate first part of the lower canaliculus. | To ensure procedure is carried out correctly. |

▶

| | | |
|---|---|---|
| **8** | Remove the dilator and carefully insert the cannula following the direction of the canaliculus to a maximum of 4–5 mm. | To ensure procedure is carried out correctly. |
| **9** | Inject the fluid slowly. Undue pressure must not be used. | To prevent damage to the lacrimal structure. |
| **10** | Warn the patient at this stage that the saline may be felt and tasted at the back of the throat. | To obtain the patient's co-operation and safety. |

**Result of the procedure**

The result will be one of several.

- The saline may pass easily into the sac, through the nasolacrimal duct and trickle into the nasopharynx. The patient will taste the saline on the back of his tongue and can be told to swallow it. The result is reported as freely patent.
- There may be partial patency with some regurgitation around the cannula.
- The saline may return through the lower punctum around the cannula. This shows an obstruction near the nasal end of the lower canaliculus.
- It may return through the upper punctum showing an obstruction in the sac or nasolacrimal duct.
- Mucopurulent discharge may return with the saline if the sac is infected. This should be reported.

The result should be reported in the notes.

Occluding the upper punctum with a second Nettleship dilator is sometimes performed if the saline has returned via the upper punctum. Syringing is repeated to try to remove the obstruction. In this case an assistant is needed to hold the dilator in place. Syringing must *not* be performed by a nurse if there is an obvious swelling over the nasolacrimal sac, as infection renders the structures more prone to damage.

The medical staff may use a set of lacrimal probes. These are used on infants in theatre, when the saline may be coloured with fluorescein to aid the detection of patency.

**3.2.14  Subconjunctival injections**

Small amounts of fluid (1.5 to 2 ml) can be injected under the bulbar conjunctiva. This form of treatment is not used as frequently as it used to be for eye infections. Here are some examples of drugs given by this method.

(1) *Mydricaine.* This contains three drugs, all having a mydriatic effect, in a 0.5 ml dose. It is used in uveitis to dilate the pupil when other methods have failed.

*Mydricaine*
| | |
|---|---|
| Atropine sulphate | 1.00 mg |
| Procaine hydrochloride | 5.00 mg |
| Adrenaline 1:1000 | 0.12 ml |

(2) *Antibiotics.* These are given subconjunctivally to treat or prevent intra-ocular infection.
| | |
|---|---|
| Cefuroxime | 100 mg in 0.5 ml water |
| Gentamicin | 10–20 mg |

(3) *Steroids.* Given to suppress the inflammatory process in cases of uveitis, steroids used include:
| | |
|---|---|
| Betamethasone | 4 mg (quick-acting) |
| Methylprednisolone | 40 mg (long-acting) |

(4) *Local anaesthetics* may be given in this manner.

**Equipment**

- Dressing pack
- Receiver with:
  - (a)  1 ml and/or 2 ml syringe(s)
  - (b)  dark green needle
  - (c)  subconjunctival needle
  - (d)  drugs for injection
- Anaesthetic drops
- Gauze squares
- Pad
- Bandage
- Tape
- Sachet of normal saline
- Steret
- Good light
- Cartella shield
- Prescribed drops or ointment (if applicable)
- Prescription/case notes
- Tissues

| Procedure | Rationale |
|---|---|
| **1** Identify the patient. (Avoid saying 'needle' is going 'into the eye'.) | To ensure the correct patient receives treatment and to obtain the patient's consent and co-operation. To reduce anxiety. |
| **2** Give prescribed analgesia (if necessary). | To reduce patient discomfort. |
| **3** Position the patient lying down or sitting in a chair with the head well supported. | To ensure patient comfort and safety. |
| **4** Commence instilling local anaesthetic drops, e.g. G. amethocaine hydrochloride 2% or G. cocaine hydrochloride 5%, one drop every five minutes over 25 minutes. | To reduce patient discomfort. |
| Cover eye with cartella shield. | To prevent damage to the cornea. |
| **5** Prepare drugs to be injected. Check with second nurse. Put subconjunctival needle on syringe firmly and check potency. | To ensure safety. |
| **6** Once eye is anaesthetised commence procedure. | For patient comfort. |
| **7** Open dressing pack as usual. | |
| **8** Clean eye if necessary. | |
| **9** Hold lower lid down and ask patient to look up. An assistant may be required. | To ensure procedure is carried out correctly. |
| **10** Hold the syringe horizontally, the needle bevel uppermost, and fingers in the correct position to inject the drug. | To ensure procedure is carried out correctly. |
| **11** Insert the needle under the conjunctiva in the folds of the lower fornix. | To ensure procedure is carried out correctly. |
| **12** Inject the drug slowly. The conjunctiva will balloon forwards as it is injected. | To ensure procedure is carried out correctly. |
| **13** On completion of the injection withdraw needle. | To ensure procedure is carried out correctly. |
| **14** Insert antibiotic ointment or drops if prescribed. | To prevent infection. |
| **15** Apply pad and bandage for four hours. | For patient comfort. |

▶

**Notes:**

- Methylprednisolone must not be mixed with any other drug.

- If no assistance is available, it may be necessary to use:
  (a)  speculum to hold the lids open;
  (b)  Moorfields forceps to hold up the conjunctiva to ease the insertion of the needle.

- Analgesics may be given before the procedure and again once the local anaesthetic has worn off.

## 3.2.15   Inserting/removing a contact lens

| Procedure | Rationale |
|---|---|

### Insertion of a lens

| | | |
|---|---|---|
| **1** Wash hands. | To prevent cross infection. |
| **2** Place contact lens on tip of index finger. | To aid insertion. |
| **3** Hold the lids apart with the other hand and ask the patient to look straight ahead. | To prevent lids blinking during insertion and to position eye correctly. |
| **4** Place the lens over the cornea. | To place in correct position. |
| **5** Ask the patient to blink. | To centre lens in correct position. |

**6** If an extended wear of bandage lens is being inserted, because they are larger, it may be necessary to evert the lower lid first and place the lens in the lower fornix. Then ask the patient to look down while you place the upper lid over the top of the lens.

### Removal of a lens

If possible ask the patient to remove his own lens. It is always easier, as people develop their own particular way of doing it.

If you have to do it:

**1** Wash your hands.

**2** (a) *Hard or gas permeable lenses:*  Place your index finger on the lens and gently move it to one side of the cornea and pull away. The eyelids can be used to lever the edge of the lens away from the cornea. A small rubber suction extractor can be used. This is squeezed between the thumb and index finger and placed on the lens. The pressure of the thumb and finger is released and the suction thus caused removes the lens with the extractor as the latter is pulled away from the eye.

(b) *Soft, extended wear and bandage lenses:*  Gently squeeze the lens between thumb and finger and remove it. Place in correctly labelled container, with normal saline solution.

### 3.2.16   Inserting/removing a prosthesis/shell

#### Inserting a prosthesis/shell

- Tell the patient what you are going to do.
- Pull up the upper lid and insert the prosthesis into the upper fornix.
- Evert the lower lid and slip lower border of the prosthesis into the lower fornix.

#### Removing a prosthesis/shell

- Tell the patient what you are going to do.
- Evert the lower lid and ease the prosthesis out. A small plastic spatula may be required to assist in the removal. The prosthesis then slips out.

### 3.2.17   Removing a dacryocystorhinostomy tube

#### Equipment

- Nasal speculum
- Stitch scissors
- Long Spencer Wells forceps
- Torch

| Procedure | Rationale |
| --- | --- |
| 1  Identify the patient. | To ensure the correct patient receives treatment and to gain the patient's consent and co-operation. |
| 2  Ask the patient to blow his nose, especially down the nostril on the affected side. | To enable the tube to be more easily removed. |
| 3  Position patient in chair. | For comfort and safety. |
| 4  Clasp the tube in the nostril with forceps. | To ensure procedure is carried out correctly. |
| 5  Cut the tube in the inner canthus. | To ensure procedure is carried out correctly. |
| 6  Pull the tube out from the nostril. | To ensure procedure is carried out correctly. |

## 3.2.18 Removing a concretion or conjunctival cyst

### Equipment

- Local anaesthetic drops
- Needle
- Good light/slit lamp
- Pad and bandage

### Procedure

**1** Tell the patient what you are going to do.

**2** Instil local anaesthetic drops.

**3** Remove concretion with the needle/puncture conjunctival cyst.

**4** If bleeding occurs from conjunctival vessels, a pad and bandage may need to be applied.

## 3.2.19 Preparing a patient for fundal fluorescein angiography

### Procedure

**1** Take visual acuity.

**2** Instil mydriatic drop to both eyes which has been written up by a doctor.

**3** Explain the procedure to the patient:
   (a) Colour photographs will be taken.
   (b) Fluorescein will be given intravenously.
   (c) The fluorescein will stain the skin yellow for about 24 hours. Urine will also be discoloured.
   (d) The patient will have to look into the camera and will be asked to look in various directions while the angiogram is being taken.
   (e) Offer tea and biscuits after procedure.

*Notes:*

- Resuscitation equipment must be at hand as fluorescein can cause analphylactic shock.

- The patient must stay for $\frac{1}{2}$ hour to 1 hour following the angiogram to enable observation for any reaction to the dye.

## 3.2.20    Preparing a patient for laser treatment

**1** Take visual acuity.

**2** Explain the procedure to the patient:
(a)  Mydriatics will be instilled if the retina is to be treated and maybe for a capsulotomy.
(b)  Local anaesthetic drops will be instilled.
(c)  The patient will have to keep his eyes very still while flashing green lights are emitted from the argon laser. Usually nothing is noted by the patient receiving laser treatment from the YAG laser.
(d)  Following capsulotomy and trabeculoplasty the intraocular pressure will be measured 1 hour after the procedure.

**3** Wipe eyes following the procedure. Lubricating jelly will have been used for the contact lens.

**4** Offer tea and biscuits.

***Note:***
Staff in the laser room should wear protective spectacles and adhere to laser safety policies.

## 3.2.21    Preparing a patient for ultra-sound

**1** Take visual acuity.

**2** Explain the procedure to the patient:
(a)  Local anaesthetic drops will be instilled.
(b)  Dilating drops will be instilled.
(c)  Keratometry will be performed prior to an A-scan.
(d)  The patient will need to look ahead and keep his eyes still while the scan is being performed.

## 3.2.22    Applying heat to the eye

Heat can be applied to the eye in several ways to reduce swelling, encourage the discharge of infected cysts, ease pain and enhance the action of drugs, especially mydriatics.

### Hot spoon bathing

A wooden spoon, covered in a suitable cloth, is dipped in hot water and held as near to the closed eye as is comfortable.

## Thermos flask

A thermos flask is filled with hot water. The head is positioned so that the steam rising from the flask bathes the closed eye.

The dangers of scalding from this and the above method must be remembered.

## The Sykes Heater

The Sykes Heater is an electrically controlled pad which is applied over the eye. It is especially useful in enhancing the action of mydriatics in uveitis.

### 3.2.23   Removal of sutures

### Equipment

- Sterile receiver with: fine scissors
  *or*
  stitch cutter
  *or*
  blade
- 1 pair fine forceps
- Normasol sachet
- Gallipot
- Dental rolls or cotton wool balls or gauze squares
- Patient's notes

| Procedure | Rationale |
| --- | --- |
| 1  Identify the patient and the site of sutures with doctor's instructions for removal. | To ensure the correct patient receives treatment at the correct site and to obtain the patient's consent and co-operation. |
| 2  Sit the patient with his head supported and in a good light. | For safety and ease of performance. |
| 3  Prepare the equipment. | |
| 4  If necessary, check with the doctor prior to the procedure. | To ensure healing has occurred. |
| 5  Clean the suture line if necessary | |
| 6  Remove the sutures. | To complete the procedure. |
| 7  Check the suture line. | To ensure it is clean and intact/healed. |

▶

| | | |
|---|---|---|
| **8** | Clear away the equipment and wash hands. | To prevent cross infection. |
| **9** | Instruct the patient on any follow-up instructions. | For continued care of the patient. |
| **10** | Record in the case notes the fact that the sutures have been removed. | For a permanent record of procedure having taken place. |

### 3.2.24   Preparing a patient and equipment for minor surgery

## Equipment

- Trolley with:
    relevant sterile instrument set
    extra instruments
    1 sheet sterile wax paper
    2 sterile linen towels or paper towels
    eye pad
    few dental rolls
    few gauze swabs
- Local anaesthetic drops
- Local anaesthetic injection
- Syringes and needles
- Mediprep
- Sutures
- Specimen pot with formaldehyde and pathology form if necessary
- Surgical gloves
- Tape

## Procedure

**1** Identify patient and check notes about the procedure to be performed.

**2** Clean and lay trolley as required.

**3** Lie the patient on couch ensuring comfort.

**4** Ensure that there is a good light source.

**5** Instil local anaesthetic drops prescribed by doctor.

**6** Prepare local anaesthetic injection.

**7** Clean around the eye with Mediprep.

**8** Assist the doctor during the procedure.

▶

9  Apply ointment/pad/bandage at the end of the procedure if necessary, which may need to be renewed before the patient goes home.

10  Explain any follow-up procedure and offer tea and biscuits.

11  Clear away the trolley and clean the instruments before re-sterilising them.

12  Complete minor operations register.

### 3.2.25  Goldmann applanation tonometry

Goldmann applanation tonometry measures the intra-ocular pressure indirectly by measuring the force necessary to flatten a 3.06 mm diameter portion of the corneal surface. The higher the intra-ocular pressure, the greater the force required.

**Measuring principle** (devised by Imbert Fick)

The cornea is flattened with a plastic prism which has a flat anterior surface and a diameter of 7.0 mm. The prism is brought into contact with the cornea by advancing the slit lamp. The measuring drum, which regulates the force applied to the pressure arm, is turned and the tension on the eyes is increased until a surface of known and constant size of 3.06 mm is flattened.

The intra-ocular pressure (in mmHg) is found by multiplying the drum reading by ten.

| Procedure | Rationale |
| --- | --- |
| 1  Ensure that the slit lamp is switched on and that the eye pieces are correctly focused. | |
| 2  Switch on the blue filter and bring into the beam of the slit lamp. | |
| 3  Adjust the angle between the illumination and the microscope to about 60°. | For accurate reading of intra-ocular pressure |
| 4  Insert the tonometer into the slit lamp base plate. The instrument can be used in either of two positions, observation is monocular with either the right or left microscope. | |
| 5  Bring the pressure arm into the notch position so that the axis of the prism and the microscope coincide. | |

▶

**Preparing the patient**

| 1 | Identify the patient. | To ensure the correct patient receives the treatment and to obtain the patient's consent and co-operation. |
| --- | --- | --- |
| 2 | Check if the patient is wearing contact lenses, if so then remove them before commencing the procedure. | Unable to perform tonometry with contact lenses in situ. |
| 3 | Instil topical anaesthesia into both eyes. | To reduce discomfort. |
| 4 | Instil fluorescein stain by means of fluorescein paper strips. | For accurate reading and to prevent too much fluorescein in the eye. |
| 5 | Instruct the patient to look straight ahead with both eyes wide open – if necessary, the patient's eyelids should be held apart by the examiner without pressure being applied to the eyeball. | For accurate measurement. |

**Measurement**

1. The prism is brought into contact with the centre of the the cornea, by advancing the slit lamp. A blue light illuminates the limbus when contact is made. The examiner looks through the microscope at this point.

2. Upon contact, a thin circular outline of fluorescein is produced. The prism splits the circle into two semi-circles coloured green. Any necessary adjustment is made by the control lever or height adjustment control on the slit lamp, until the flattened area is seen as two semi-circles of equal size in the middle of the field of view.

3. The pressure on the eye is increased by manually adjusting the measuring drum on the tonometer, until the inner borders of the two fluorescein rings just touch each other open. The inner border of the ring represents the demarcation between the cornea flattened by application and the cornea not flattened.

4. The amount of force required to do this is translated by the scale into a pressure reading of mmHg, which is found by multiplying the drum reading by ten.

Tonometry can also be performed using the handheld Perkins' tonometer or a tonopen.

### 3.2.26   Keratometry

Keratometry is used to measure the greater and lesser curvatures of the cornea, usually in conjunction with biometry, to discover the strength of the intra-ocular lens required by a patient following cataract extraction. As biometry involves contact with the eye which may distort it slightly, keratometry should be performed before biometry.

Each eye is tested separately. There are a number of machines used but the principles of each are similar. The patient should be sat comfortably with his chin and forehead on the rests and asked to look down the barrel of the keratometer. The patient must keep as still as possible. The nurse looks through the eyepieces and may need to adjust the machine until she sees the cornea clearly and certain points that must be aligned before a reading can be taken.

### 3.2.27 Biometry

This uses an A-scan to measure the axial length of the eye. As a probe touches the eye, a local anaesthetic must be instilled in the patient's eye. The patient is positioned comfortably with his chin supported on a rest such as a slit lamp and asked to fix his gaze. The nurse must also ensure that she is comfortable and within easy reach of the foot plate. Once the patient's eye is aligned, the nurse gently places the probe on the cornea. A steady hand is required as the probe must make contact to measure correctly. Excess pressure however will indent the cornea and give a false reading which the nurse must be able to identify.

By measuring both eyes a comparison can be made to further prove accuracy as it is unusual to find a marked difference between the axial length of the two eyes.

It may be easier to obtain a reading after the pupil has been dilated.

The information gained from the keratometry and biometry is fed into a computer, which produces the desired intra-ocular lens power for the individual patient.

### 3.2.28 Perimetry

This is performed to assess the degree of peripheral and central visual loss. Again there are different machines in use but the principles are similar. The patient must be made comfortable as the procedure can take a long time. The patient is asked to position his chin and forehead on the rests and to fixate on a target. One eye is tested at a time, the other eye being covered. The patient indicates that he can see various lights being presented to him either verbally or by pressing a buzzer. Most machines are computerised, the result appearing on a printout. The majority of patients having perimetry are elderly and need to be encouraged to perform the task as their concentration may not be very good.

# 4 The Globe: a Brief Description

## 4.1 INTRODUCTION

This chapter is deliberately brief to avoid repetition, as more detailed descriptions can be found in the individual chapters on each structure. Its aim is to enable you to see the interrelations of the various structures.

The globe is situated in the bony *socket* or *orbit* (see Section 5.1), which affords it protection. Also in the socket are nerves, muscles, blood vessels and fat.

The globe is also protected by the upper and lower *eyelids* (see Section 5.2), which contain muscles, secretory glands and eyelashes.

The *lacrimal gland* (see Section 6.2) sits in the upper outer aspect of the frontal bone of the orbit and produces tears. These tears drain into the *lacrimal drainage system* (see Section 6.3). This is composed of an upper and lower punctum situated on the inner aspects of the upper and lower lid margins, the upper and lower canaliculi and the lacrimal sac, which opens into the nasal duct.

There are six extra-ocular muscles (see Section 13.1), which move the eye in the direction of gaze. There are four recti muscles and two oblique muscles.

The *conjunctiva* lines the lid and overlies the sclera, terminating at the cornea. The *globe* or *eyeball* (Fig. 4.1) is approximately 2.5 cm in diameter by the age of 3 years. It has three layers.

(1) The *outer protective layer* comprises the *sclera* (see Section 8.2) for approximately its posterior four-fifths and the *cornea* (see Section 8.1) for its anterior one-fifth. The cornea is clear to allow light rays through and is highly sensitive. The sclera is composed of tough white fibrous tissue.

(2) The *middle layer* is the pigmented vascular *uveal tract* (see Chapter 9). The *choroid* forms approximately the posterior four-fifths and the *ciliary body* and *iris* the anterior one-fifth. The iris is a diaphragm allowing varying amounts of light to enter the eye through the pupil in its centre. The ciliary processes produce aqueous and the ciliary muscles control the shape of the lens for focusing. The

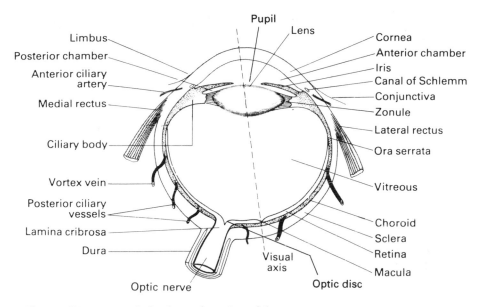

Fig. 4.1 Diagrammatic horizontal section of the eye.

choroidal blood vessels supply the underlying outer layers of the retina.

(3)   The *inner layer* is formed by the *retina* (see Section 12.1) and is the nerve ending layer containing rods and cones, which receive the light stimulus that is sent via the optic nerve to the occipital cortex for interpretation.

*Aqueous* (see Section 10.5) is produced by the ciliary processes, which are part of the ciliary body, and flows into the posterior chamber, through the pupil, into the anterior chamber and drains through the trabecular meshwork and the canal of Schlemm in the angle of the anterior chamber. It nourishes the lens and cornea.

The *anterior chamber* (see Section 10.3) is the area between the cornea and the iris.

The *posterior chamber* (see Section 10.4) is the area between the posterior surface of the iris and the anterior surface of the lens.

The *lens* (see Section 11.1) is suspended by the suspensory ligaments from the ciliary body and lies behind the iris. It is clear to allow light rays to pass through and changes shape so light rays can be focused on the retina for near vision.

*Vitreous* (see Section 12.3) is a gelatinous substance, which fills the posterior segment of the eye between the lens and the retina.

## 4.2   THE NERVE SUPPLY TO THE EYE

- The *oculomotor* or third cranial nerve supplies the:
  - (a)   levator palpebral superioris muscle
  - (b)   superior rectus muscle
  - (c)   inferior rectus muscle
  - (d)   medial rectus muscle
  - (e)   inferior oblique muscle

  Its branch, the short ciliary nerve supplies:
  - (a)   the sphincter muscle of the iris
  - (b)   the ciliary muscle.
- The *trochlea* or fourth cranial nerve supplies the superior oblique muscle.
- The *trigeminal* or fifth cranial nerve. The first division of the trigeminal nerve is the *ophthalmic division*. This division has three branches:
  - (1)   *lacrimal*, supplying the lacrimal gland;
  - (2)   *frontal*, supplying the skin of the forehead;
  - (3)   *nasociliary*
    - (i)    infratrochlea supplying the inside of the nose;
    - (ii)   long ciliary supplying the dilator muscle of the iris, the conjunctiva and the cornea.
- The *abducens* or sixth cranial nerve supplies the lateral rectus muscle.
- The *facial* or seventh cranial nerve supplies the orbicularis muscle.

## 4.3   THE BLOOD SUPPLY TO THE EYE

The *ophthalmic* artery and its branches supply the blood to the eye and it is drained by the *ophthalmic* vein and its branches.

- The *central retinal* artery and vein supply and drain the retina.
- The *short posterior ciliary* artery and *choroidal* vein supply and drain the choroid.
- The *long posterior ciliary* artery supplies the ciliary body.
- The *anterior ciliary* artery supplies the:
  - (a)   ciliary body
  - (b)   conjunctiva
  - (c)   corneal limbus.
- The *arterial circle of iris* is formed from:
    the *long posterior ciliary* artery
    the *anterior ciliary* artery
  and supplies the iris.
- The *anterior ciliary* vein drains the:
  - (a)   ciliary body
  - (b)   iris

(c)    conjunctiva

(d)    corneal limbus.

- The *conjunctival* artery and vein supply and drain the conjunctiva.
- The *superior* and *inferior medial palpebral* artery and vein supply and drain the:

(a)    conjunctiva

(b)    eyelids

(c)    lacrimal sac.

- The *episcleral* artery and vein supply and drain the sclera.
- The *lacrimal* artery and vein supply and drain the:

(a)    lacrimal gland

(b)    eyelids.

- The *supra-orbital* artery and vein supply and drain the upper eyelids.
- The *muscular* artery and vein supply and drain the extra-ocular muscles.
- The *nasal* artery and vein supply and drain the lacrimal sac.
- The *frontal* artery and vein supply and drain the forehead.
- The four *vortex* veins drain the ciliary body, iris and choroid leaving the globe at its equator to drain into the *ophthalmic* vein.

# 5 The Protective Structures

## 5.1 THE ORBIT

The eyeball or globe is protected by the bony socket or orbit in which it sits (Fig. 5.1).

The orbit is composed of seven bones:

(1)  maxilla
(2)  frontal
(3)  lacrimal
(4)  ethmoid
(5)  sphenoid
(6)  zygomatic
(7)  palatine

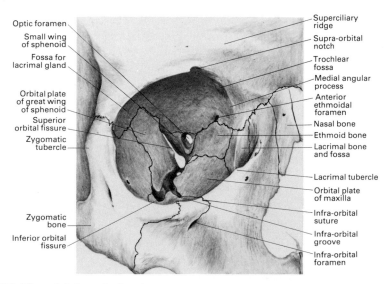

Optic foramen
Small wing of sphenoid
Fossa for lacrimal gland
Orbital plate of great wing of sphenoid
Superior orbital fissure
Zygomatic tubercle
Zygomatic bone
Inferior orbital fissure

Superciliary ridge
Supra-orbital notch
Trochlear fossa
Medial angular process
Anterior ethmoidal foramen
Nasal bone
Ethmoid bone
Lacrimal bone and fossa
Lacrimal tubercle
Orbital plate of maxilla
Infra-orbital suture
Infra-orbital groove
Infra-orbital foramen

**Fig. 5.1** The orbit from in front.

Each orbit has four walls; a floor, roof, lateral wall and medial wall. The two medial walls are parallel to each other and the two orbits diverge to allow for a greater field of vision. The orbits are pyramid-shaped with the apex posteriorly.

### 5.1.1 Areas of the orbit

- *Roof* – triangular-shaped and made up of the frontal bone anteriorly and part of the sphenoid posteriorly.
- *Floor* – triangular-shaped and made up of the maxilla anteriorly, part of the zygomatic laterally and the palatine posteriorly.
- *Lateral wall* – composed of the zygomatic anteriorly and the sphenoid posteriorly.
- *Medial wall* – composed of four bones; from the front backwards: part of the maxilla, the lacrimal, the ethmoid and part of the sphenoid.
    Three apertures are situated at the apex of each orbit:

(1)  The *optic foramen* through which passes:
     (a)  the optic nerve (second cranial nerve) leaving the orbit (see optic pathways, Section 12.2.1);
     (b)  the ophthalmic artery entering the orbit, running underneath the optic nerve.
(2)  The *superior orbital fissure* through which pass:
     (a)  nerves:
          (i)   oculomotor (third cranial nerve) – superior and inferior branches;
          (ii)  trochlea (fourth cranial nerve);
          (iii) trigeminal (fifth cranial nerve) – three branches of the first division (ophthalmic division): lacrimal; frontal; nasociliary;
          (iv)  abducens (sixth cranial nerve);
     (b)  blood vessels: ophthalmic vein – superior and inferior branches.
(3)  The *inferior orbital fissure* through which pass:
     (a)  the infra-orbital artery;
     (b)  the trigeminal nerve – some branches of the second division (maxillary division).

Surrounding the globe in the socket are muscles, ligaments, blood vessels, nerves and fat. *Tenons capsule* is a thin membrane which encircles the globe from the margin of the cornea to the optic nerve, adhering closely to the sclera beneath it.

## 5.2   THE EYELIDS

The functions of the eyelids are to protect the globe and to lubricate its anterior surface (Fig. 5.2). The top lid, the larger of the two, closes over the globe to protect it. By blinking, the tear film is spread over the anterior surface thus lubricating it (see Sections 6.4.3 and 6.4.4).

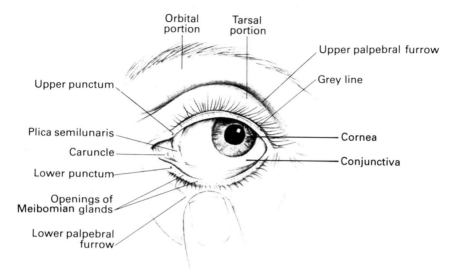

**Fig. 5.2**  The outer appearance of the eye and eyelid.

### 5.2.1   Areas of the lid (Fig. 5.3)

* *Palpebral conjunctiva* lining the undersurface.
* *Tarsal plate* – a band of connective tissue lying posteriorly forming a stiff plate.
* *Skin* on the outer surface.
* *Grey line* – intermarginal sulcus, where the skin joins the palpebral conjunctiva on the lid margin.
* *Hair follicles* – lashes, near the grey line.
* *Fat* – surrounding the structures.
* *Glands.*
    (a)  *Meibomian glands.* There are 20–30 Meibomian glands in each lid, contained within the tarsal plate, their ducts opening through the palpebral conjunctiva just behind the lashes. They produce a sebaceous substance which creates the oily layer of the tear film (see Section 6.4).
    (b)  *Glands of Moll.* These are sweat glands producing sebum.
    (c)  *Glands of Zeis.* These are modified sebaceous glands which open into the lash follicles.

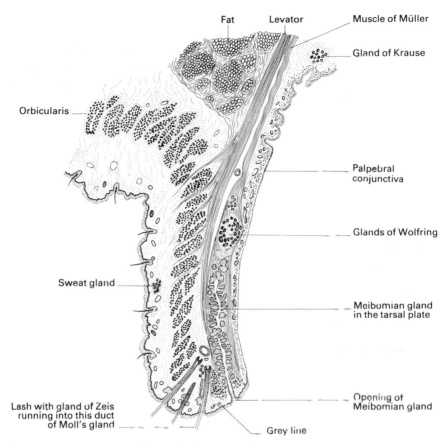

Fat    Levator    Muscle of Müller

Gland of Krause

Orbicularis

Palpebral
conjunctiva

Glands of Wolfring

Sweat gland

Meibomian gland
in the tarsal plate

Opening of
Meibomian gland

Lash with gland of Zeis
running into this duct
of Moll's gland

Grey line

**Fig. 5.3** Vertical section through the upper lid.

(d)  *Glands of Krause and Wolfring.* These are situated in the fornices. They are accessory tear glands.
(e)  *Sweat glands.* These open directly onto the skin of the outer surface.
- *Muscles.* There are three muscles supplying the eyelid.
  (a)  *Orbicularis:*
    (i)   origin – lacrimal bone;
    (ii)  insertion – deep in the fascia around the lacrimal sac;
    (iii) function – to close the lids and to screw up the eyes;
    (iv)  nerve supply – facial nerve (seventh cranial nerve).
  (b)  *Levator palpebral superioris:*
    (i)   origin – Annulus of Zinn (a ring tendon surrounding the optic nerve at the apex of the orbit);
    (ii)  insertion – into the tarsal plate, palpebral ligaments and skin of the upper lid;

(iii)  function – to lift the upper lid;
(iv)   nerve supply – oculomotor (third cranial nerve).
(c)  *Müller's muscle.* This is a smooth muscle:
(i)    origin – in the levator palpebral superioris muscle;
(ii)   insertion – tarsal plate;
(iii)  function – to provide extra elevation to the upper lid;
(iv)   nerve supply – sympathetic nervous system.

### 5.2.2  Sensory nerve supply

- Upper lid: ophthalmic division of the trigeminal nerve (fifth cranial nerve).
- Lower lid: maxillary division of the trigeminal nerve.

### 5.2.3  Blood supply

The blood supply to and drainage from the eyelids is v˙a:

- lacrimal artery and vein;
- supra-orbital artery and vein (upper lid);
- superior and inferior medial palpebral artery and vein.

## 5.3  CONDITIONS OF THE ORBIT

### 5.3.1  Orbital cellulitis

Orbital cellulitis (Fig. 5.4) is an acute purulent inflammation of the cellular tissue of the orbit. It is an ophthalmic emergency because of optic nerve compression. It is more common in children and is usually unilateral.

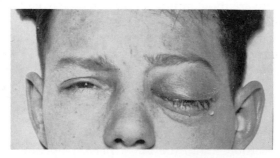

**Fig. 5.4** Orbital cellulitis.

## Causes

- Spread of infection from neighbouring structures, e.g. nasal sinus.
- Sepsis following penetrating injuries.
- Following septic operations, e.g. enucleation.
- Facial erysipelas.
- Spread of pyaemia – causative organisms: *Pneumococcus*; *Staphylococcus*; *Streptococcus*.

## Signs

- Proptosis of the affected eye, pushed forward by the inflamed tissue within the orbit, behind the eyeball.
- Red and inflamed lids.
- Chemosis of conjunctiva.
- An abscess may form over the upper eyelid.

## Patient's needs

- Admission to hospital if necessary
- Relief of symptoms:
  - (a) pain – especially on eye movement;
  - (b) fever – there may be rigors;
  - (c) anorexia;
  - (d) general malaise.

## Nursing action

- Admit patient to ward if necessary.
- Give prescribed analgesia for pain. Local heat application may be comforting.
- Fan and/or tepid sponge patient to bring down temperature.
- Administer prescribed antibiotics:
  - (a) oral, e.g. ampicillin 500 mg 4 times a day;
  - (b) eyedrops, e.g. G. chloramphenicol, gentamicin, 2–4 hourly;
  - (c) in severe cases, intravenous antibiotics may be prescribed.
- Give nourishing fluids and a light diet.
- General nursing care of an ill patient.
- Dress abscess if this forms.
- Prepare for, and give, post-operative care of patient following drainage of abscess sinuses.

## Complications

- The infection may spread backwards into the brain causing:

    (a)   cavernous sinus thrombosis;
    (b)   meningitis;
    (c)   brain abscess.
- Panophthalimitis may occur.
- Sinus formation, if the cause is a sinusitis.
- Optic atrophy due to pressure on the nerve.

If orbital cellulitis occurs in a child, he is usually referred to an ear, nose and throat specialist, as the cause is invariably from the nasal cavity.

### 5.3.2   Preseptal cellulitis

Preseptal cellulitis is often preceded by infection of the teeth or sinuses or by trauma. The infection does not spread beyond the orbital septum of the upper lid into the orbit. The signs and symptoms are similar to orbital cellulitis but the condition is not so dangerous.

### 5.3.3   Cavernous sinus thrombosis

The cavernous sinus is situated near the pituitary gland. Through it pass many of the veins draining structures around the face, including the orbit, globe, nose, mouth, sinuses and the meninges. Thus infection can spread from any of these structures into the cavernous sinus. It may also spread from a general infectious disease or septic focus elsewhere in the body. It is a serious condition. 50% of cases are bilateral.

### Signs

Signs are as for orbital cellulitis, plus some others.

- Paralysis of the extra-ocular muscles, as their nerves pass through the cavernous sinus and are thus involved.
- Dilated pupil(s), usually non-reactive due to the trigeminal nerve being involved as it also passes through the cavernous sinus.
- Anaesthetic cornea due to the involvement of the trigeminal nerve.
- Reduced visual acuity due to pressure.
- Papilloedema due to pressure.
- Signs of cerebral irritation may also be present.

### Patient's needs and nursing action

- These are as for orbital cellulitis.
- The antibiotics will be administered by the intravenous route in large doses.
- Anticoagulants may be prescribed.

### 5.3.4 Thyrotoxic exophthalmos

Graves' disease describes the most common cause of hyperthyroidism and is thought to be due to an autoimmune problem. It usually affects women between the ages of 20 and 45 who have signs and symptoms of thyrotoxicosis together with ophthalmic signs. Ophthalmic signs can occur in patients who are clinically euthyroid and in these cases the disease is referred to as ophthalmic Graves' disease. The signs and symptoms tend to be similar.

### Signs

- *Exophthalmos.* Unilateral or bilateral. Inflammatory exudates and plasma cell infiltration of the orbital fat and extra-ocular muscles push the globe forwards (Fig. 5.5).
- *Lid lag.* When looking downwards, the top lid normally moves with the eye. In this condition, the lid moves very slowly down or not at all. This is possibly due to sympathetic overactivity of Müllers muscle.
- *Lid retraction.* The upper lid retracts, giving the typical 'stare' associated with thyroid eye disease. The sclera above the cornea is visible. This is probably due to involvement of the levator muscle.
- *Corneal exposure.* Corneal exposure occurs because:
  (a) the lids are unable to close over the protruding globe;
  (b) defective blinking occurs because of involvement of the lid muscles.

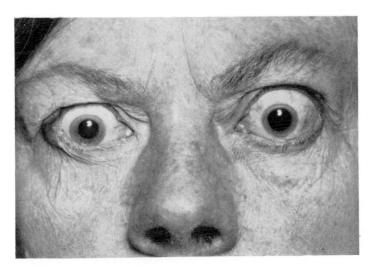

**Fig. 5.5** Mild exophthalmos.

- *Exophthalmoplegia.* Exophthalmoplegia is the inability to move the eye in the fields of gaze because the extra-ocular muscles are involved due to infiltration and later fibrosis. Diplopia results.
- In hyperthyroidism, signs of thyrotoxicosis such as tachycardia and muscular tremors may be present.

## Patient's needs

- Protection of the exposed cornea is the most important factor.
- Prevention of complications, which can result in loss of vision.
- Investigation and treatment of thyroid state by an endocrinologist.
- Correction of diplopia.
- Treatment of lid lag.
- In severe cases, rapid relief of orbital pressure.

## Nursing action

- *Corneal exposure.* The nurse will:
  (a)  instruct the patient in application of ointment such as simple eye ointment or chloramphenicol at night;
  (b)  prepare the patient for a tarsorrhaphy, which may be necessary; the edges of the eyelids are sewn together, usually in the lateral aspect, to protect the cornea;
  (c)  instruct the patient in the use and care of a bandage contact lens. This is a large contact lens which covers the whole of the cornea, thereby giving protection (see Appendix 2).
- Explain the investigations needed for thyroid function estimations.
- Explain to the patient that diplopia can be treated by wearing glasses with prisms in the lenses. Squint operation may be carried out when the thyroid state is stable.
- Treatment for lid lag. The nurse will prepare the patient for lid surgery when Müller's muscle will be divided.
- In severe cases where emergency treatment is required to reduce the orbital pressure, the nurse will:
  (a)  give the prescribed high doses of systemic steroids;
  (b)  prepare the patient for orbital decompression; part of the lateral wall of the orbit is removed so the orbital contents can prolapse and therefore relieve the pressure on the optic nerve;
  (c)  prepare the patient for radiotherapy.

## Complications

- Corneal ulceration due to exposure keratitis.
- Visual loss due to optic nerve compression, central retinal artery and vein occlusion.

- Cataract formation due to metabolic disturbance to the lens.
- Secondary glaucoma due to compression on the globe by the orbital contents, causing the intra-ocular pressure to rise.

## 5.4 CONDITIONS OF THE EYELIDS

### 5.4.1 Chalazion

A chalazion is a swelling of one of the Meibomian glands due to a blockage of its duct (Fig. 5.6). It can affect either the upper or lower lid. It may become infected, when it is sometimes called an *internal hordeolum*. Staphylococci are commonly the cause of the infection. The swelling may fluctuate in size during the course of the condition. Some chalazions point to the skin surface. Some people appear to be prone to this condition and should be examined to ensure that they are not diabetic. Some chalazions are so large as to obstruct vision and, by pressing on the cornea, cause astigmatism.

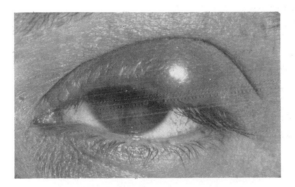

**Fig. 5.6** Meibomian cyst.

### Patient's needs

- Relief of swollen eyelid, which is causing pain and discomfort.
- Relief of sticky discharge, which may be present.

### Nursing action

- Instruct the patient to apply steam to the eye (see Section 3.2.22).
- Instruct the patient in the use of the antibiotic ointment which will be prescribed if the chalazion is infected. Chloramphenicol is the usual ointment. This is used 3 to 4 times a day after the eye has been steamed. This should be continued for 7–10 days.

- Instruct the patient to keep the eyelids clean by using warm water to wash off any crusts and discharge twice a day.
- Instruct the patient to return if the swelling does not subside, as the simple operation of incision and curettage can be performed once the infection has cleared up, to remove any remaining material.

### 5.4.2   Oedema of the lids

Oedema of the lids is a common condition and, because of the looseness of the tissue, the swelling can be so great as to close the eye.

### Causes

- Insect bites/stings.
- Dermatitis.
- Stye.
- Chalazion.
- Associated with:
    orbital cellulitis;
    conjunctivitis;
    dacryocystitis;
    drug allergy (Fig. 5.7).

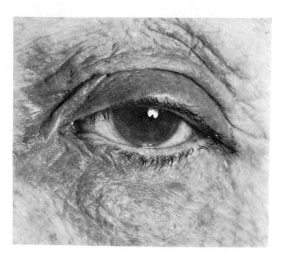

**Fig. 5.7** Atopic irritation.

### Patient's needs

- Reduction of swelling.
- Treatment of cause.

**Nursing action**

- Explain to the patient methods to reduce the swelling:
  (a)  cold compress;
  (b)  bathing eyelid in sodium bicarbonate solution.
- Explain to him the treatment of the cause of the condition. Antihistamine ointment and/or tablets may be used to treat insect bites/stings.

### 5.4.3  Blepharitis

Blepharatis can be an acute or a chronic inflammatory condition of the lid margins and is usually bilateral (Fig. 5.8). Blepharitis is often undetected, even when eyes have been examined for other reasons (Bonner *et al.* 1994).

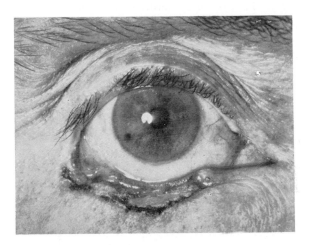

**Fig. 5.8** Staphylococcal blepharitis.

**Causes**

- Staphylococcal – chronic infection.
- Seborrhoeic – excessive secretion of lipid from Meibomian glands.
- It may be associated with dandruff, poor hygiene, eczema or allergy to make-up, or drugs.
- Acne rosacea.

**Signs**

- Red, swollen lid margins.
- Scales on lashes.

**Patient's needs** (see Advice Sheet No. 1)

- Relief of symptoms:
  (a)   itchiness around eye;
  (b)   discharge if an infective cause;
  (c)   burning sensation.


**Nursing action**

- Instruct patient on the treatment.
  (a)   Use clean, warm, face cloth over eyelids.
      (i)    Clean lid margin and lashes with dilute baby shampoo or dilute sodium bicarbonate ($\frac{1}{2}$ teaspoon to $\frac{1}{2}$ cup of cooled, boiled water) twice a day.
      (ii)   Application of antibiotic ointment along the lid margin 2 or 3 times a day, if prescribed.
  (b)   *Dandruff.* Treatment of dandruff in head hair with antidandruff shampoo.
  (c)   *Make-up.* Stop using make-up or change the brand used.
  (d)   *Eczema.* May be treated with steroid ointment.
  (e)   *Drugs.* Stop offending drug.
  (f)   *Poor hygiene.* Instruct patient on improving general hygiene, especially to hair, face and hands.
- Inform patient that the treatment will need to continue for several weeks, if not for life, as it is a chronic condition although the frequency of treatment can be reduced. Encourage him not to give up the treatment, even if it does not appear to be working in the initial stages.


**Complications**

Complications can occur following blepharitis caused by infective organisms that results in ulceration of the lid margin.

- Conjunctivitis.
- Trichiasis and its sequelae due to chronic ulcerations, which, when healed, contract the skin in that area, causing the lash(es) to turn inwards.
- Entropion or ectropion of the lower lid in particular.
- Corneal ulcer.


**5.4.4   Stye or external hordeolum**

A stye or external hordeolum is an inflammation of a gland of Zeis which opens into the lash follicle. An abscess forms, which usually points near an eyelash (Fig. 5.9).

**ADVICE SHEET No. 1**
**Eye Casualty Department**

# BLEPHARITIS

Blepharitis is an inflammatory condition of the eyelids. Oils and other products normally secreted by the eye build up on the lid surface and eyelashes, resulting in symptoms of eye irritation and redness. Though we often use a combination of many forms of treatment, including antibiotic tablets and antibiotic ointments, the mainstay of treatment is careful cleaning of the eyelids and lashes to remove the irritating substances.

To obtain the best results, please follow the instructions listed below, preferably twice a day. Remember blepharitis is a skin condition that may be with you for a lifetime. The treatment is aimed at minimising your symptoms and making you more comfortable. Regular lid hygiene should become a part of your daily routine.

### (1) Warm compresses

Soak a clean facecloth in water as warm as the lids can stand and then apply it to the closed lids for a period of 5 to 10 minutes. You may need to rewarm the cloth repeatedly. This will not only feel good, but will make the lid oils easier to remove.

### (2) Lid cleaning

Following the warm compresses, clean the eyelid margins with a clean moistened cotton wool bud, using a side to side motion. This will remove the debris from the eyelids and eyelashes. If debris remains, as often happens in the early days of treatment, use the cotton wool bud to scrub between the lashes. The cotton wool bud may be moistened with a little baby shampoo.

### (3) Application of ointment

If an ointment has been prescribed by your doctor, this should be applied following the warm compresses and lid scrubs. Place a small amount of ointment on your fingertips and rub it into the lid margin and lashes. 6 mm ($\frac{1}{4}$" of ointment should be placed inside the lower eyelid and this treatment is conveniently carried out at bedtime.

Having followed the steps outlined above, we expect the redness and irritation to have improved within two to eight weeks of starting treatment. To stop treatment altogether will probably result in a recurrence of problems, so use it with the minimum frequency during the week to keep the eyelids comfortable.

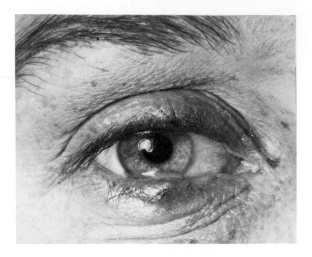

**Fig. 5.9** An external stye.

## Signs

- Swelling, often with pointing on the lid margin situated near a lash.

## Patient's needs

- Relief of pain and swelling.

## Nursing action

- Explain the treatment, which is similar to that for a chalazion (see Section 5.4.1).

Incision and curettage is not necessary for a stye. Removal of the affected lash will cause the abscess to drain, but this action is momentarily very painful.

If styes recur, the patient should be investigated for diabetes mellitus.

### 5.4.5   Meibomianitis

Meibomianitis is an uncommon condition affecting elderly patients. It is a bilateral chronic inflammation of the Meibomian glands. It may be caused by acne rosacea.

## Signs

- Red, swollen lids.

**Patient's needs**

- Relief of symptoms:
  (a)  irritation;
  (b)  stinging;
  (c)  discharge.

**Nursing action**

- Instruct the patient to:
  (a)  clean the eye with warm water;
  (b)  apply the ointment to the lids, e.g. chlortetracycline 3 times a day;
  (c)  massage the lids to promote drainage.
- Explain to the patient that the treatment may necessarily be prolonged.

### 5.4.6  Trichiasis

Trichiasis is a condition in which the lashes grow inwards and rub on the cornea. This may follow, for example, blepharitis, trauma or surgery to the lids. Often the cause is unknown.

**Patient's needs**

- Removal of the offending lash(es) which is(are) causing irritation to the eye.

**Nursing action**

- Remove the lash by:
  (a)  epilating it using epilation forceps (see Section 3.2.7). This will need to be repeated regularly;
  (b)  assisting the doctor to use electrolysis, when an electrode is introduced to each offending lash follicle to destroy it:
    (i)   prepare local anaesthetic injection and drops;
    (ii)  instil antibiotic ointment to the eye following the procedure.
  (c)  assisting the doctor to apply cryotherapy (liquid nitrogen) to the lash follicle to destroy it:
    (i)   prepare local anaesthetic injection and drops;
    (ii)  instil antibiotic ointment following the procedure, e.g. betamethasone;
    (iii) warn the patient that the eye will be uncomfortable for a few days following cryotherapy.
  (d)  assisting the doctor to apply argon laser (Yung *et al.* 1994) to the offending lash.
- Check the cornea for abrasions from the ingrowing lash(es) by staining

it (them) with G. fluorescein. If these have occurred, instruct the patient to use the prescribed antibiotic ointment 3 times a day for 3 or 4 days.
- Instruct the patient to return for further lash epilation as soon as he feels that the eye is becoming irritated, so that complications can be avoided by prompt treatment.

### Complications

- Corneal abrasions.
- Corneal ulceration.
- Superficial corneal opacities.
- Vascularisation of the cornea.

Unfortunately, treatment is rarely completely successful and usually needs to be repeated at regular intervals.

### 5.4.7   Entropion

Entropion is the turning inwards of the eyelid, usually the lower lid (Fig. 5.10).

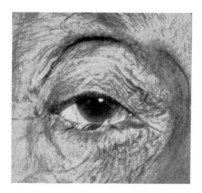

**Fig. 5.10** Spastic entropion.

### Causes

- Spastic entropion occurring in old age when spasm of the orbicularis muscle occurs, causing the lid to turn inwards.
- Cicatricial contraction of the palpebral conjunctiva following trauma or disease to the lid or conjunctiva.

### Patient's needs

- Relief of symptoms of irritation in the eye.

**Nursing action**

- Strap the lower lid to pull it outwards (see Section 3.2.10).
- Prepare the patient and equipment for surgery to evert the lid. Care must be taken when performing entropion surgery to avoid an ectropion resulting.
- Entropion operations include:
  - (a) cautery;
  - (b) transverse lid everting suture;
  - (c) Wies procedure – lid splitting and marginal rotation;
  - (d) Fox procedure – excision of triangle of conjunctiva and tarsal plate;
  - (e) shortening of lower lid retractors.

**Complications**

The complications for entropion are the same as those for trichiasis.

### 5.4.8   Ectropion

Ectropion is the turning outwards of the eyelid, usually the lower lid (Fig. 5.11).

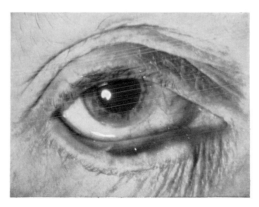

**Fig. 5.11** Ectropion.

**Causes**

- Senile ectropion due to relaxation of the orbicularis muscle, turning the eyelid outwards.
- Cicatricial ectropion due to scarring following trauma or chronic disease of the lid or conjunctiva, pulling lid outwards.
- Paralytic ectropion occurring with palsies of the seventh cranial nerve.

Because the punctum is not in apposition to the bulbar conjunctiva when an ectropion is present, the tears cannot flow through the punctum and into the lacrimal drainage system. They therefore spill over the lid margin and down the cheek.

## Patient's needs

- Relief of symptoms:
  (a)  watering eye;
  (b)  irritable sensation;
  (c)  discharge, which may be present;
  (d)  sore skin area over maxilla from constantly wiping away tears.

## Nursing action

- Prepare the patient and equipment for surgery to invert the lid:
  (a)  Lazy-T procedure – full thickness excision;
  (b)  retropunctal cautery;
  (c)  Bick procedure – full thickness excision.

Care must be taken when performing ectropion surgery to avoid an entropion resulting.

### 5.4.9   Ptosis

Ptosis is drooping of the upper lid. It may be unilateral, bilateral, constant or intermittent.

## Causes

- *Congenital ptosis* (Fig. 5.12). Caused by failure of development of the levator muscle. It is usually bilateral. The child with bilateral congenital ptosis has to tilt his head backwards to be able to see properly. This will prevent amblyopia developing (see Section 13.3.2). There is a danger that amblyopia will occur with unilateral ptosis.
- *Acquired ptosis*. Caused by:
  (a)  mechanical failure – abnormal weight on lid due to oedema, tumour, scarring;
  (b)  muscle involvement – trauma to muscle. Disease involving muscles, e.g. muscular dystrophy, myasthenia gravis. If, following an injection of neostigmine, the ptosis is temporarily relieved, myasthenia can be diagnosed;
  (c)  paralysis of nerves supplying the upper lid.

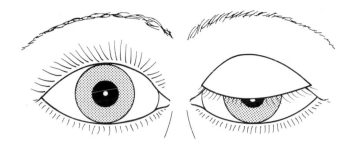

**Fig. 5.12** Left ptosis.

## Patient's needs

- Correction of lid, if it obscures sight.
- Treatment of underlying disease.

## Nursing action

- Explain and prepare the patient for any of the following treatments:
  - (a) lid surgery to resect the levator muscle or remove growths if present;
  - (b) wearing of special glasses or contact lenses with 'ptosis edge' to hold the lid up;
  - (c) treatment of causative or underlying disease, e.g. myasthenia gravis.

### 5.4.10 Blepharospasm

This is a condition that causes forceful, painful spasm eyelid closure resulting in difficulty in opening the eye. Photophobia is present and the condition is exacerbated by bright lights, stress and excessive movement around the person. It can cause the individual concerned to become socially isolated and unable to work. There may be some accompanying contraction of the lower facial muscles. Treatment is by injections of *Botulinum* (Osaka & Keltner 1991) into the orbicularis muscle. This is repeated every 2 to 3 months.

### 5.4.11 Tumours

Growths on the eyelids can be either benign or malignant.

### Benign

- Papilloma
- Warts

- Granulomas
- Xanthelasma

## Malignant

- Basal cell carcinoma (see Fig. 5.13)
- Squamous cell carcinoma
- Melanoma

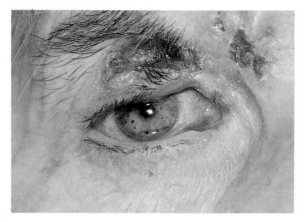

**Fig. 5.13** Rodent ulcer (basal cell carcinoma).

## Patient's needs

- Removal of tumour, especially if it is thought to be malignant.

## Nursing action

- Prepare the patient and equipment for removal of the tumour. Skin grafting or flaps may be necessary depending on the size and position of the tumour.
- Send specimen to the laboratory for histology.

Surgery to the lids must be performed with great care to avoid either an ectropion, entropion or trichiasis resulting.

# 6 The Lacrimal System and Tear Film

## 6.1 INTRODUCTION

The lacrimal system (Fig. 6.1) consists of:

- the lacrimal gland;
- the lacrimal drainage system comprising:
  - (a) the puncta;
  - (b) the canaliculi;
  - (c) the lacrimal sac;
  - (d) the nasolacrimal duct.

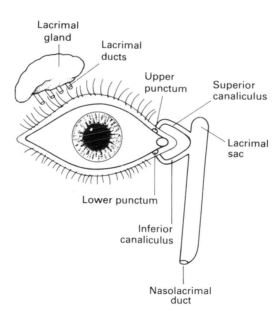

**Fig. 6.1** Lacrimal system. (Reprinted from Darling & Thorpe *Ophthalmic Nursing* (1981), Fig. 36, p. 144 by permission of the publisher Baillière Tindall Limited, London.)

## 6.2  THE LACRIMAL GLAND

The lacrimal gland is situated in the upper, outer quadrant of the orbit, in the lacrimal fossa of the frontal bone. It is almond-shaped and is divided into two lobes by the levator palpebral muscle:

(1)  the superior or orbital lobe;
(2)  the inferior or palpebral lobe.

There are 10 to 12 drainage channels leaving the lacrimal gland to convey tears to openings in the upper fornix.

### 6.2.1  Blood supply

The lacrimal artery and vein supply and drain blood to and from the lacrimal gland.

### 6.2.2  Nerve supply

Nerve supply to the lacrimal gland is via the lacrimal nerve, the first branch of the ophthalmic division of the trigeminal nerve.

### 6.2.3  Function of the lacrimal gland

The function of the lacrimal gland is to produce tears in response to stimulation of the trigeminal nerve through, for example, emotion, foreign body in the eye, or obnoxious fumes, such as smoke or peeled onions.

## 6.3  THE LACRIMAL DRAINAGE SYSTEM

### 6.3.1  The puncta

The upper and lower puncta are small round or slightly oval apertures situated on the lid margin on a slight elevation called the lacrimal papilla. This is a pale area, due to the presence of few blood vessels, about 6 mm from the inner canthus. Both puncta are normally turned inwards towards the bulbar conjunctiva so tears can drain into them. They are surrounded by fibres of the orbicularis muscle.

### 6.3.2  The canaliculi

The upper and lower canaliculi are narrow ducts passing from each puncta vertically for 1.5–2.0 mm, which then turn medially and travel horizontally for 10 mm. They usually unite to form a common canaliculus for about 1 mm before opening out into the lacrimal sac.

### 6.3.3   The lacrimal sac

The lacrimal sac is situated in the lacrimal fossa of the lacrimal bone, being a blind-ended sac superiorly, 5 mm wide and 12–14 mm in length. Fibres of the orbicularis and Horner's muscles surround the sac.

### 6.3.4   The nasolacrimal duct

The nasolacrimal duct is a downward continuation of the sac for 12–24 mm before opening into the inferior meatus of the nose beneath the inferior turbinate bone.

All the passages of the lacrimal drainage system are lined with epithelium.

### 6.3.5   Blood supply

Blood is supplied to and drained from the nasolacrimal duct via:

- nasal artery and vein;
- superior and inferior medial palpebral artery and vein.

### 6.3.6   Nerve supply

The infratrochlear nerve, a branch of the nasociliary nerve which is the third branch of the ophthalmic division of the trigeminal nerve, provides the nerve supply for the nasolacrimal duct.

### 6.3.7   Lymphatic drainage

Lymph is drained from the nasolacrimal duct via the submaxillary nodes.

## 6.4   THE TEAR FILM

The tear film is a mixture of secretions from the accessory tear glands of Krause and Wolfring, the goblets cells of the conjunctiva and the Meibomian glands of the eyelids. The tear film is a constant film of fluid bathing the conjunctiva and cornea. Excess tears are produced by the lacrimal gland.

### 6.4.1   Three layers of the tear film (Fig. 6.2)

(1)  *Oil.* The outer layer, produced by the Meibomian glands of the eyelids, it prevents evaporation and spillage of tears over the lid margin.

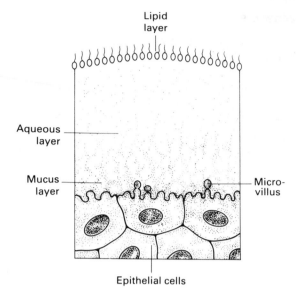

Lipid
layer

Aqueous
layer

Mucus
layer

Micro-
villus

Epithelial cells

**Fig. 6.2** Three layers of the tear film. (Reproduced with permission from Vaughan, D.G. & Asbury, T. (1983) *General Ophthalmology* (10th edn), Appleton & Lange.)

(2)  *Aqueous.* The middle layer, the 'tears proper', produced by the glands of Krause and Wolfring.
(3)  *Mucin.* The inner layer, produced by the goblet cells of the conjunctiva, is a wetting substance for easy spread over the cornea.

### 6.4.2  Composition of tears

95–98%  Water
  2–5%   Protein
         Glucose
         Urea
         Sodium
         Potassium
         Chloride
Lysozyme – an antimicrobial enzyme.
Immunoproteins and antimicrobial agents.
Normal pH is 7.1–8.6 (Saude 1992).

### 6.4.3  Function of tears

• Refraction – to provide an optically smooth surface to the cornea.
• Lubrication of the front of the eyeball.
• Cleansing action by washing away dust particles from the eye.
• Protection from infection by secreting the enzyme lysozyme and immunoproteins and antimicrobial agents.

### 6.4.4   Flow of tears

Tears flow across the front of the eyeball into the lacrimal drainage channels as a result of the following factors.

- Blinking. Lid movements assist the flow of tears across the front of the cornea and conjunctiva.
- Capillary attraction into the puncta and canaliculi.
- The lacrimal pump. The contraction of orbicularis and Horner's muscles around the puncta and lacrimal sac dilate these structures and draw in the tears.
- Gravity assists the tear flow downwards through the channels.

## 6.5   CONDITIONS OF THE LACRIMAL SYSTEM

### 6.5.1   Dacryoadenitis

Dacryoadenitis is a rare acute or chronic inflammation of the lacrimal gland.

**Causes**

- *Acute:*
  (a)   complication of: mumps; measles; influenza; or conjunctivitis;
  (b)   gonorrhoea, syphilis;
  (c)   following injury to the lacrimal gland.
- *Chronic:*
  (a)   sarcoidosis;
  (b)   tuberculosis;
  (c)   lymphatic leukaemia;
  (d)   lymphosarcoma.

**Signs**

- Swelling of the upper lid, especially in the temporal aspect (Fig. 6.3).
- S-shaped curve to the upper lid.

**Patient's needs**

- Relief of pain.
- Admission to hospital if condition is severe.
- Incision of abscess where necessary.
- Treatment of active infection.
- Treatment of underlying cause, if possible.

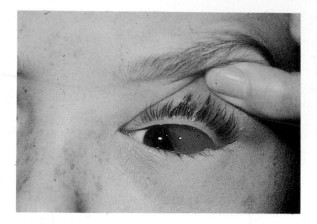

**Fig. 6.3** Dacryoadenitis.

**Nursing action**

- Admit patient to hospital if condition is severe.
- Give/instruct the patient:
    (a)    to instil antibiotic drops and ointment for 7–10 days;
    (b)    to take oral antibiotic if the condition is severe;
    (c)    to take analgesics.
- Apply local heat for pain relief.
- Prepare patient and equipment for incision of abscess.

**6.5.2   Dacryocystitis**

Dacryocystitis is an acute or chronic inflammation of the lacrimal sac (Fig. 6.4). It is more common than dacryoadenitis. It is usually unilateral and follows obstruction to the lacrimal drainage system.

**Causes**

- *Acute:*
    (a)    most are unknown;
    (b)    following chronic dacryocystitis;
    (c)    causative organisms – staphylococci, streptococci, pneumococci.

- *Chronic:*
    (a)    following trauma to the lacrimal system;
    (b)    following chronic conjunctivitis, e.g. trachoma.

- *Infant.* Failure of canalisation of lacrimal ducts following birth.

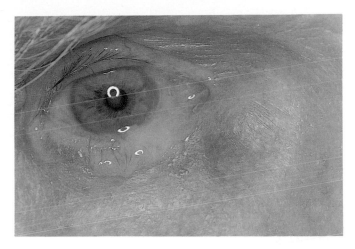

**Fig. 6.4** Dacryocystitis.

## Signs

### Acute and infant

- Swelling over lacrimal sac.
- Pus regurgitating through punctum.
- Conjunctivitis.
- Watering eye.

### Chronic

- May be swelling over lacrimal sac, which can be recurrent.
- Watering eye.

## Patient's needs

### Acute

- Relief of pain, which can be severe, discharge and watering eye.

### Chronic

- Relief of watering eye due to blockage of drainage channels.
- Diagnosis and treatment of obstruction.

### Infant

- Relief of pain, discharge and watering eye.
- Admission to hospital for probing of ducts if initial treatment fails.

**Nursing action**

*Acute*

- Apply/instruct the patient how to apply warm compress to the inflamed area.
- Give/instruct him to take the prescribed analgesia and antibiotics, e.g. tetracycline 250 mg 4 times a day for 7–10 days.
- Clean/instruct him how to clean the eye if sticky and instil prescribed antibiotic drops and ointment.

*Chronic*

- Perform lacrimal sac washout to detect area of blockage (see Section 3.2.13). **Note:** This is never carried out on a patient with an acute infection of the sac as the inflamed walls are easy to perforate.
- Prepare patient for dacryocystogram. This is an X-ray using radio-opaque dye, which is introduced into the lacrimal drainage system to show up any blockage. Warn the patient that it is an uncomfortable procedure and that he should be accompanied home following this test as he may feel unwell.
- Admit and prepare the patient for surgery to correct the blockage. Dacryocystorhinostomy is performed to open up a new drainage channel into the nasal cavity. Sometimes a tube is left *in situ* for 3–6 months to maintain the patency of the new drainage channels.
- Post-operative care:
  (a) clean the eye and suture line;
  (b) instil antibiotic drops;
  (c) remove sutures 5–7 days post-operatively (usually in out-patient department);
  (d) if a tube is present, instruct the patient not to blow his nose vigorously as this will dislodge the tubing;
  (e) remove the tubing in 3–6 months' time in outpatient department (see Section 3.2.17).

*Infant*

- Instruct the mother to instil local antibiotic drops, e.g. G. chloramphenicol.
- Instruct the mother to massage over the lacrimal sac area to remove accumulated mucus which may lead to a patent duct.
- Admit the child to the ward if the above methods fail to open the canaliculus.
- Give pre-operative care prior to probing of the ducts, which is performed under a general anaesthetic.
- Give post-operative care: instil antibiotic drops.

## Complications

Following acute dacryocystitis fistula formation may develop. Dacryo-cystorhinostomy is not always successful in curing the watering eye.

### 6.5.3 Epiphora

Epiphora is watering of the eye.

#### Causes

- Acute or chronic dacryocystitis (see above).
- Ectropion (see Section 5.4.8).
- A small or tight punctum.
- Increased secretion of tears due to reflex stimulation of the lacrimal gland, e.g. by wind, smoke, onions, or a foreign body in the eye.

#### Patient's needs

- Dilation of a small or tight punctum.
- Removal of causative agent of increased stimulation.

#### Nursing action

- If a foreign body is present, remove this (see Section 3.2.9).
- If the cause is a small or tight punctum, this needs to be dilated reg-ularly over a period of several months. This is usually performed every week or so using a Nettleships dilator, holding it in place in the punctum for 5 minutes.
- Prepare patient and equipment for a 1, 2 or 3 snip operation, which will be carried out if the dilation fails. During this procedure, per-formed under local anaesthetic, 1, 2 or 3 snips are made behind the punctum to release the muscle around the punctum.

### 6.5.4 Dry eye syndrome (keratoconjunctivitis sicca)

Dryness of the eye results from any disease associated with deficiency of any of the layers of the tear film. Its name (dry eyes) implies a non-sig-nificant condition. This is not the case. In addition to being very uncomfortable, it has the potential to be sight threatening.

#### Causes

*Oil deficiency*

- Exposure: proptosis, facial palsy.
- Hot, dry climate/environment.

- Lid damage.
- Blepharitis.
- Meibomianitis.

## Aqueous deficiency

- Sjögren's syndrome (arthritis, dry eye, achlorhydria).
- Removal/absence of glands.
- Trachoma.
- Chronic dacryoadenitis.
- Drugs: beta blockers, diuretics.
- Old age/menopause.

## Mucin deficiency

- Trachoma.
- Chemical burns.
- Chronic conjunctivitis.
- Antihistamines.
- Stevens–Johnson syndrome.
- Xerophthalmia.

## Other causes

- Deficient blinking.
- Corneal scarring.

## Signs

- Usually a normal-looking eye.
- Dead corneal and conjunctival epithelial cells show up when stained with Rose Bengal 1% drops (not used very often now).
- Damaged epithelial, corneal and conjunctival cells stain with fluorescein drops.
- Breaks in the tear film are seen when stained with G. fluorescein.

## Patient's needs (see Advice Sheet No. 2)

- Relief of symptoms which include:
  - (a)  gritty feeling;
  - (b)  itching;
  - (c)  burning sensation;
  - (d)  inability to produce tears;
  - (e)  pain around and in the eye;

(f)   sometimes a red eye;

(g)   difficulty in opening eyes on waking and moving lids;

(h)   watering eye. If the outer oil layer of the tear film is deficient, tears will spill over the lower lid margin.

- Investigation and treatment of underlying cause, if possible.
- Treatment with replacement tears.

---

**ADVICE SHEET No. 2**
**Eye Casualty Department**

# DRY EYES

**What are dry eyes?**

In order to stay healthy and comfortable, your eyes need to be covered by a thin film of tears. The tears are produced by tear glands and are spread over the surface of the eye when you blink. In some people these tears are produced in very small amounts, or are of poor quality. The result is that small patches of the front of the eye dry out, causing irritation, redness and excessive blinking (and even, paradoxically, watering in some people).

**Why do I have dry eyes?**

This is a very common condition and usually no cause can be found. Occasionally it is associated with other conditions which may need to be excluded.

**Is it serious?**

Although it can be uncomfortable, the condition is not serious.

**What can I do about it?**

Your doctor will suggest that you use some form of artificial tears, such as hypromellose drops. These can usually be bought in any chemist without prescription whenever your eyes become uncomfortable. You may have to use the drops very frequently (even hourly) and often a lubricating ointment at night. Avoid dry, smoky atmospheres. If your house or office is centrally heated, ensure the atmosphere does not get too dry. House plants, humidifiers or saucers of water on radiators may help.

**Nursing action**

- Perform tear production test (see Section 3.2.11).
- Instruct the patient to use the prescribed artificial tears, e.g. hypromellose. These drops can usually be used as often as the patient requires, to keep the eye feeling comfortable, and will probably need long-term use.
- Cautery to the punctum or insertion of punctal plugs may be employed to prevent what little tears are produced from draining into the punctum.

**Complications**

- Chronic conjunctivitis due to loss of the protective function of the tear film and lysozyme.
- Corneal scarring and vascularisation.
- Corneal ulceration, thinning and perforation.
- Eventual loss of the eye through recurrent infections.

# 7 The Conjunctiva

## 7.1 INTRODUCTION

The conjunctiva is a thin, transparent mucous membrane lining the upper
and lower lids and covering the globe up to the limbus.

### 7.1.1 Areas of the conjunctiva

There are three areas to the conjunctiva.

- *Palpebral conjunctiva* – lines the upper and lower lids.
- *Bulbar conjunctiva* – reflects back to cover the sclera up to the limbus.
- *Fornices* – the upper and lower fornices are blind sacs, formed where
  the bulbar and palpebral conjunctiva fold back over each other.

### 7.1.2 Layers of the conjunctiva

- *Epithelial layer* – contains the goblet cells.
- *Stromal layer* – contains the blood vessels, nerves and the glands of
  Krause and Wolfring (in upper only).

The conjunctiva is connected to Tenon's Capsule around the limbus.
Elsewhere it is loosely attached, especially in the fornices where there are
folds of the conjunctiva. This allows for easy mobility of the eyeball.

### 7.1.3 Functions of the conjunctiva

- Allows easy movement of the eyeball.
- Goblet cells provide mucin for the tear film.
- It is a protective layer to the eyeball by being a physical barrier and by
  its rich blood supply.

### 7.1.4 Blood supply

There is a rich blood supply, especially in the fornices, delivered and
drained via:

- anterior ciliary artery and vein;
- superior and inferior medial palpebral artery and vein;
- conjunctival artery and vein.

### 7.1.5   Nerve supply

The nerve supply to the conjunctiva is by the long ciliary branch of the nasociliary nerve from the trigeminal nerve.

### 7.1.6   Lymphatic drainage

Lymphatic drainage is through the pre-auricular, parotid and sub-maxillary nodes.

## 7.2   CONDITIONS OF THE CONJUNCTIVA

### 7.2.1   Conjunctivitis

Conjunctivitis is inflammation of the conjunctiva, which has several causes:

- bacterial
- viral
- allergic
- chlamydial
- fungal
- parasitic
- associated with other diseases
- other ophthalmic conditions
- mechanical

**Bacterial conjunctivitis**

Bacterial conjunctivitis can be either acute or chronic.

*Causative organisms*

*Streptococcus*
*Staphylococcus aureus*
*Pneumococcus*
*Gonococcus*
Haemolytic *Streptococcus*

*Signs*

Typically there is conjunctival injection, especially in the fornices where the blood supply is rich (Fig. 7.1). The eye may, on the other hand, be white or only mildly red. Discharge is variable, but typically is present in the mornings, and on waking the eye is difficult to open because the eyelids are stuck together. This is a very important point when taking a history from a patient with suspected conjunctivitis. The eyelids may be red and inflamed. The condition may be unilateral or bilateral.

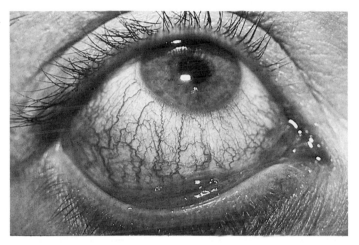

**Fig. 7.1** Bacterial conjunctivitis. (Reproduced with permission from Khaw, P.T. & Elkington, A.R. (1985) Disorders of the external eye, *The Practitioner*, **229**, 317.)

**Patient's needs** (see Advice Sheet No. 3)

- Relief of symptoms:
  (a)  grittiness – often a foreign body sensation; the patient may think something has got into the eye;
  (b)  sticky eye.
- Treatment to clear discharge.
- Instructions on treatment and prevention of spread.

*Nursing action*

- Take swab from affected eye for culture and sensitivity if severe. A Gram stain may also be taken.
- Clean the eye(s) and instruct the patient on cleaning it(them), using cooled, boiled water.
- Instruct him to instil drops which will be prescribed if the condition

---

**ADVICE SHEET No. 3**
Eye Casually Department

# CONJUNCTIVITIS

Conjunctivitis is an infection of the white part of the eye. It is not serious but can be contagious: ensure that you use your own flannel, soap and towel. Wash your hands before and after instilling your eye drops. If the infection spreads to the other eye use the drops in that eye as well. If the eyes are sticky bathe them with cool water which has been boiled.

Do not use the drops on anyone else.

The infection should resolve within 1–2 weeks. If it does not do so please ring the Casualty Department for further advice.

**Further advice & instructions**

. . . . . . . . . . . . . . . . . . . . . . . . . . . . . . . . . . . . . . . . . . . . . . . . . . . . . . . . . .

. . . . . . . . . . . . . . . . . . . . . . . . . . . . . . . . . . . . . . . . . . . . . . . . . . . . . . . . . .

. . . . . . . . . . . . . . . . . . . . . . . . . . . . . . . . . . . . . . . . . . . . . . . . . . . . . . . . . .

. . . . . . . . . . . . . . . . . . . . . . . . . . . . . . . . . . . . . . . . . . . . . . . . . . . . . . . . . .

---

is severe. This is usually chloramphenicol drops, which may be prescribed 2-hourly for 2 days and then 4 times a day for 3–5 days.
- Instruct patient on how to prevent the infection spreading either to his other eye or to other members of the household.
  (a)   Wash hands before and after instilling drops and ointment.
  (b)   Use separate face flannels and towels in the home, as this is the usual method of spread of infection.
- Warn him never to wear a pad over the eye, as it provides a suitable environment for further bacterial growth.

## Ophthalmia neonatorum

Severe conjunctivitis occurring in a baby less than 28 days old is a notifiable disease. This may be caused by *Gonococcus*, *Streptococcus*, or *Chlamydia* which is the most common cause.

## Signs

- Severe discharge.
- Red, swollen eyelids (Fig. 7.2).
- Chemosis.
- Unilateral or bilateral infection.

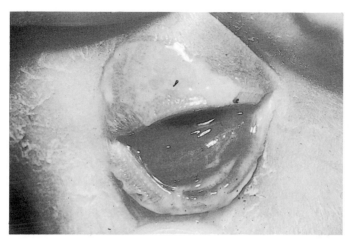

**Fig. 7.2** Ophthalmia neonatorum.

## Nursing action

- Take swabs from baby's eye(s). A swab may also need to be taken from the mother's vagina.
- Lay the baby on the affected side if the condition is unilateral, to prevent it spreading to the other eye.
- Clean/instruct the mother to clean the eye(s) as often as is necessary.
- Instil/instruct the mother to instil the prescribed antibiotics.
  - (a) Drops: e.g. gentamicin, hourly initially; penicillin may also be instilled hourly initially. The frequency of administration will be reduced as the condition improves.
  - (b) Ointment: e.g. gentamicin at night.
  - (c) Oral antibiotics.
- If the mother has a vaginal infection, this will be treated with antibiotics.

## Complications of chronic conjunctivitis

- Conjunctival scarring.
- Chronic blepharitis due to upset in the tear film.

- Conjunctival ulceration leading to perforation due to decreased conjunctival nutrition.
- Marginal corneal ulcer.

**Viral conjunctivitis**

*Causes*

- Adenovirus.
- Measles.
- Varicella.
- Herpes simplex (see Section 8.5.3).
- *Chlamydia.*

*Signs*

- Red/pink eye (Fig. 7.3).
- Chemosis, if severe.
- Follicles may be present on the palpebral conjunctiva.
- Cornea – superficial punctate keratitis.
- Enlarged pre-auricular nodes, which may be tender.
- Bleeding from conjunctival vessels in severe adenoviral conjunctivitis.

*Patient's needs*

- Relief of symptoms:
    (a)   watering eye;

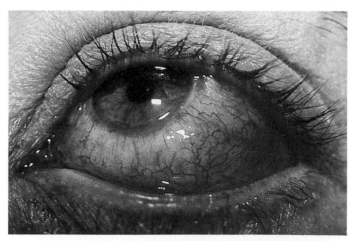

**Fig. 7.3** Adenoviral conjunctivitis. (Reproduced with permission from Khaw, P.T. & Elkington, A.R. (1985) Disorders of the external eye, *The Practitioner*, **229**, 317.)

(b) irritation, which may be present;
(c) photophobia;
(d) generally unwell feeling.
- Instruction on treatment.

## Nursing action

- Take a swab for viral studies if requested.
- Usually no treatment is given as viral infections are self-limiting, running a course of 7–10 days.
- Drugs:
  (a) Hypromellose may be prescribed for patient comfort.
  (b) Steroids may be given in severe or recurrent attacks, but must be given with care (see Section 17.6.1).
- Advise the patient that wearing dark glasses will help the photophobia.

## Allergic conjunctivitis

*Causes*

- *Hay fever* – tends to be seasonal.
  (a) Signs:
      (i) severe chemosis;
      (ii) red eye;
      (iii) papillae may be present on the palpebral conjunctiva.
  (b) Symptoms:
      (i) irritation of the eye;
      (ii) watering eye;
      (iii) nasal signs of hay fever may be present.
  (c) Treatment:
      (i) antihistamines such as xylometazoline hydrochloride (Otrivine Antisin) drops 4 times a day;
      (ii) G. sodium cromoglycate (Opticron) 2% 4 times a day;
      (iii) steroids, if condition is severe.
- *Vernal conjunctivitis or spring catarrh* (Fig. 7.4) – common, seasonal warm-weather condition, some patients being affected annually in the spring or early summer. It usually affects the 10–14 years age group, boys more than girls.
  (a) Signs: giant papillae on subtarsal conjunctiva, called 'cobblestones'. Corneal punctate epithelial erosions.
  (b) Symptoms: irritation, foreign body sensation in the eye.
  (c) Treatment:

       (i)    G. sodium cromoglycate 2%. Steroids, if severe;

       (ii)   test for allergy and avoid cause, if possible.

- *Eczema:*
  - (a) Signs:
    - (i)    redness of eye;
    - (ii)   red, dry, scaly eyelid;
    - (iii)  skin around eye may be affected;
    - (iv)  slight discharge may be present;
    - (v)   fine papillae on palpebral conjunctiva.
  - (b) Symptoms:
    - (i)    burning sensation;
    - (ii)   photophobia.
  - (c) Treatment:
    - (i)    antibiotic drops to prevent secondary infection;
    - (ii)   steroid cream, e.g. betamethasone or sodium phosphate or hydrocortisone to eyelid and affected skin around the eye.
- *Phlycten* – a small, yellow nodule in the conjunctiva or cornea. It can grow onto the cornea and may rupture and cause an ulcer. It is thought to be caused by an allergy to *Staphylococcus aureus* bacteria or a virus. It tends to occur in undernourished children and those living in poor conditions and is not so common nowadays.
  - (a) Signs: yellow phylcten with engorged blood vessels surrounding it.
  - (b) Symptoms:
    - (i)    a foreign body sensation;
    - (ii)   photophobia.
  - (c) Treatment:
    - (i)    antibiotic drops and ointment;
    - (ii)   steroid drops;
    - (iii)  dark glasses for photophobia.

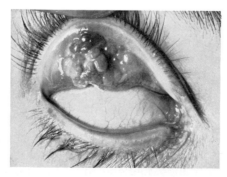

**Fig. 7.4** Spring catarrh.

*Complication*

Keratitis is the complication of allergic conjunctivitis.

**Chlamydia trachomatis**

There are two types of disease caused by different serotype of *Chlamydia trachomatis*:

(1)  *Chlamydia* or adult inclusion conjunctivitis (TRIC – trachoma inclusion conjunctivitis) is caused by serotypes D to K. It typically affects young adults, with eye symptoms appearing a week after sexual activity.
(2)  Trachoma is caused by serotypes A, Ba and C. It is common in hot, dry climates where there is a low standard of hygiene and flies are abundant.

   The disease runs a long and chronic course. The incubation period is 5–14 days. In a child, the onset is insidious, but it is acute in an adult.

*Signs*

*   Red eye.
*   Discharge.
*   Follicles and papillae on palpebral conjunctiva.
*   Chemosis of bulbar conjunctiva.
*   Small tender pre-auricular nodes.
*   Keratitis.
*   Pannus formation on upper portion of the cornea. This is the development of new blood vessels growing into the cornea. It is usually a later sign of the disease.

*Patient's needs*

*   Relief of symptoms:
    (a)  pain;
    (b)  photophobia;
    (c)  watering eye.
*   Instruction on treatment.

*Nursing action*

*   Take swab for testing for *Chlamydia* ensuring sufficient material is obtained (see Section 3.2.6). The sub-tarsal area needs to be swabbed.
*   Prepare equipment for doctor to take conjunctival scrapings for *Chlamydia* tests.

- Instruct the patient on the treatment:
    - (a)  Oc. chlortetracycline 1% 4 times a day for 6 weeks;
    - (b)  oral tetracycline 250 mg 4 times a day for 6 weeks;
    - (c)  sulphonamides may also be given.

## Complications

- Conjunctival scarring and fibrosis resulting in:
    - (a)  blockage to the drainage of the accessory tear glands and lacrimal gland resulting in a reduced tear film;
    - (b)  reduction in secretion of mucin.

      **Both (a)** and **(b)** will cause a reduction in lysozyme in the tear film and therefore the patient will be prone to chronic conjunctivitis;
    - (c)  blocked lacrimal ducts from conjunctival scarring, which could cause dacryocystitis;
    - (d)  entropion and trichiasis;
    - (e)  ptosis, due to scarring under the top lid.
- Scarring of the cornea due to pannus formation, trichiasis and scarred palpebral conjunctiva.

## Treatment of the complications

- Scarred conjunctival tissue can be treated by expressing and curetting the follicles. Plastic surgery may be necessary to correct lid deformities.
- Corneal graft to replace the scarred cornea. This can only be performed once the lid deformities have been corrected so that they will not abrade the grafted cornea.
- Administration of replacement teardrops to treat the dry eyes.
- Use of antibiotic drops for chronic bacterial conjunctivitis.
- Antibiotic treatment for dacryocystitis.
- A dacryocystorhinostomy to correct the blocked nasolacrimal ducts.

## Fungal conjunctivitis

Fungal conjunctivitis is caused by *Candida albicans*. Babies can be affected during birth through an infected birth canal. Fine white plaques are apparent on the conjunctiva. Affected adults have blepharitis.

The treatment is with nystatin drops and ointment.

## Parasitic conjunctivitis

In hot climates, parasites causing onchoceriasis, or river blindness, and schistosomiasis, or bilharzia, can induce conjunctivitis.

## Conjunctivitis caused by other diseases

General diseases which cause conjunctivitis are:

- Skin diseases:
  - (a) psoriasis
  - (b) pemphygoid
  - (c) acne rosacea
  - (d) pemphigus.
- Sjögren's syndrome (Section 6.5.4)
- Thyroid disease.
- Reiter's syndrome.

## Ophthalmic conditions causing conjunctivitis

- Dacryocystitis.
- Canaliculitis.
- Dry eyes.

The treatment is that of the general disease or ophthalmic condition.

## Mechanical conjunctivitis

Conjunctivitis can occur after the conjunctiva has been exposed to:

- wind;
- fumes;
- smoke;
- dust;
- dirt particles;
- chemicals.

## 7.2.2 Subconjunctival haemorrhage

Subconjunctival haemorrhage occurs as a result of blunt or penetrating injury (see Chapter 14) but it can also occur spontaneously or as a result of a sudden increase in pressure in the eye, as occurs with violent sneezing or heavy lifting. The subconjunctival blood vessels burst, the affected area varying in size; in severe cases it can cover the whole of the sclera causing swelling, but usually sparing the superior aspect as it pools inferiorally from gravity. In cases occurring spontaneously, the patients usually have few symptoms apart from a dull ache. It is a condition that looks more severe than it is. It can be a sign of hypertension, vascular disease or a blood clotting disorder.

**Patient's needs**

- Location of the cause, if any, of spontaneous haemorrhage.

**Nursing action**

Ask the patient if he had exerted any undue pressure before the hae-morrhage occurred, e.g. by heavy digging in the garden, sneezing fit, rubbing the eye.

- Test a specimen of urine; if abnormal, inform the doctor.
- Take the blood pressure; if abnormal, inform the doctor.
- Reassure the patient that the haemorrhage will not cover the cornea.
- Inform him that it may spread further before it begins to resolve and that it may take 2–3 weeks to clear completely, similar to a bruise. Usually there is no specific treatment.

### 7.2.3  Pterygium

A pterygium is a triangular-shaped nodule in the conjunctiva (Fig. 7.5), usually occurring on the nasal side, but it can be temporal. It usually occurs in people who live in hot, dry climates or who work in the open air. It is a degenerative process and can encroach on the cornea. If it affects the vision, it can be removed under local anaesthetic. Beta rays or cytotoxic eyedrops can be given following removal to prevent recurrence.

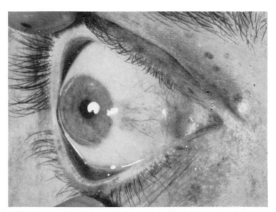

**Fig. 7.5** Pterygium.

### 7.2.4  Pinguecula

A pinguecula is a yellow, triangular nodule found in the conjunctiva of the elderly and in people who work in exposed conditions. It affects the nasal side and later the temporal side. It does not spread to the cornea and no treatment is necessary unless it becomes inflamed, when steroid drops will reduce the condition. It can be removed for cosmetic reasons.

### 7.2.5 Concretions

Concretions are white deposits found in the conjunctiva. They are fairly common and are usually symptomless. Occasionally they are large enough to give a foreign-body sensation, when they can be removed under local anaesthetic (see Section 3.2.18). If bleeding occurs during this procedure, a pad and bandage should be applied.

### 7.2.6 Conjunctival cysts

Cysts can occur in the conjunctiva. If they cause symptoms, they are easily punctured under local anaesthetic (see Section 3.2.18). This can be a recurrent condition.

# 8 The Cornea and Sclera

## 8.1 INTRODUCTION

The cornea and sclera comprise the outer, protective layer of the eyeball. The cornea forms the anterior one-fifth and the sclera the posterior four-fifths.

## 8.2 THE CORNEA

The cornea is a transparent structure which fits into the surrounding sclera like a watchglass. It is convex, avascular and highly sensitive.

### 8.2.1 Measurements

Vertical       10.6 mm
Horizontal    11.5 mm
Thickness      0.6 mm centrally
               1.0 mm peripherally.

The thinness of the cornea must be remembered when removing corneal foreign bodies.

### 8.2.2 Five layers of the cornea (Fig. 8.1)

(1) *Epithelium.* There are 5–6 layers of epithelial cells, which are continuous with the conjunctival epithelium. The basement membrane is the innermost layer of the epithelium. This is the only layer of the cornea that regenerates following trauma.
(2) *Bowman's membrane.* A layer of connective tissue.
(3) *Stroma.* This comprises 90% of the cornea. It is composed of parallel connective tissue.
(4) *Descemet's membrane.* A layer of elastic fibres.
(5) *Endothelium.* A single layer of endothelial cells.

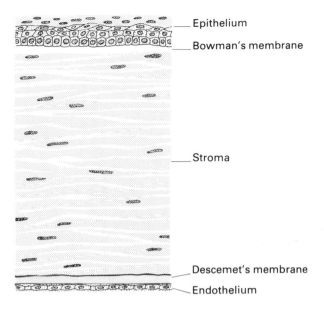

**Fig. 8.1** Transverse section of the cornea.

### 8.2.3   Function of the cornea

- Protection.
- Refraction of light. The convex shape of the cornea allows most of the refraction of light rays within the eye to take place here, approximately 40 dioptres. The cornea must remain transparent to allow light rays to enter the eye and for sight to be clear. There are three reasons for this clarity.
  - (a) Avascularity of the structure. No blood vessels impede the transmission of light rays.
  - (b) Uniform structure of the stromal layer. The fibres lie in a parallel fashion. If they are pushed apart, for example by oedema, the structure becomes opaque and blurred vision results.
  - (c) Dehydration. The cornea is kept dehydrated by the endothelial layer. This is a sodium pump whereby sodium, and therefore water, is pumped out of the cornea to be replaced by potassium. Where this layer is damaged the pump ceases to work efficiently.

### 8.2.4   Blood supply

The blood supply and drainage is via the anterior ciliary artery and vein by limbal diffusion.

The cornea also receives some nourishment from aqueous and the tear film.

### 8.2.5   Nerve supply

The cornea is highly sensitive, receiving its nerve supply from the long ciliary nerve of the nasociliary nerve. This is the third branch of the ophthalmic division of the trigeminal nerve. The nerve endings lie under the epithelial layer.

## 8.3   THE SCLERA

'Sclera' in Greek means 'hard'. The sclera is the 'white' of the eye, composed of dense, white, non-uniform collagen fibres. It is kept hydrated and is, therefore, opaque. The sclera extends from the cornea (the limbus) to the optic nerve.

It is 0.6–1.00 mm thick, although where the four recti muscles are inserted into it, it is only 0.3 mm thick.

It has a protective function.

### 8.3.1   Areas of the sclera

There are four areas to note.

- *Lamina cibrosa* – a sieve-like structure where a few strands of scleral tissue pass behind the optic disc.
- *Posterior aperture* – lies around the optic nerve and is the area where the long and short ciliary vessels and nerves penetrate the sclera to travel forward in the eye to supply the choroid and ciliary body.
- *Four middle apertures* – situated at the equator where the four vortex veins exit through the sclera.
- *Anterior aperture* – lies 4 mm posterior to the limbus where the anterior ciliary vessels puncture the sclera.

### 8.3.2   The limbus

The limbus is the transitional zone 1.2 mm wide between the cornea, conjunctiva and sclera.

### 8.3.3   The episclera

The episclera is a fine elastic tissue covering the surface of the sclera. It has a rich blood supply from the long posterior ciliary arteries to nourish the sclera lying beneath it.

### 8.3.4   Scleral nerve supply

The ciliary nerve from the oculomotor nerve provides the nerve supply to the sclera.

## 8.4   PHYSIOLOGY OF CORNEAL SYMPTOMS

- Pain – due to many pain fibres being present in the cornea.
- Blurred or reduced vision – due to a lesion obstructing light rays entering and refracting at the cornea.
- Photophobia and watering – due to irritation of the corneal nerve endings.

## 8.5   CONDITIONS OF THE CORNEA

### 8.5.1   Exposure keratitis

Exposure keratitis is an inflammation of the cornea resulting from drying of the cornea because the eyelids cannot protect it adequately. It is potentially a dangerous condition as, without treatment, it can lead to ulceration and perforation of the cornea.

The lids are unable to cover the cornea either because of proptosis of the eyeball or the inability of the lids to move over the eyeball. Once recognised, this condition must be treated promptly with measures being taken to protect the cornea. Bandage contact lenses can be used or a tarsorraphy performed plus the use of eye ointment to form a protective layer. Botulinum injections are given to induce a ptosis to cover the cornea (Kirkness *et al.* 1985).

### 8.5.2   Corneal ulcers

(1)   *Hypopyon ulcer.* This usually occurs in the elderly, being caused by a bacterium (Fig. 8.2). The hypopyon may be sterile, occurring as a result of severe uveitis.

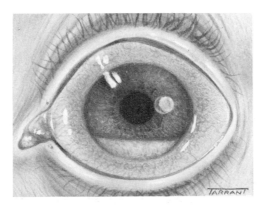

**Fig. 8.2** Corneal ulcer with hypopyon.

(2)  *Marginal ulcer.* This can be caused by a bacterium and can also be associated with acne rosacea and chronic conjunctivitis. Again they are commoner in the elderly.

 If they do not heal, a *ring ulcer* may form as multiple marginal ulcers join together. Ring ulcers can be associated with collagen disease.

(3)  *Mooren's ulcer* is a rare condition of unknown cause, affecting mainly elderly, debilitated people. The edges of the ulcer overhang, giving a 'cliff-hanging' appearance. They are extremely difficult to treat.

## Signs

- Red eye.
- Hypopyon may be present.

## Patient's needs

- Relief of symptoms:
  (a)  severe pain;
  (b)  foreign body sensation;
  (c)  lacrimation;
  (d)  photophobia;
  (e)  reduced visual acuity.
- Antibiotic treatment to the eye.

## Nursing action

- Prepare equipment and patient for corneal scrape.
- If the condition is severe and/or the patient is elderly, admit him to hospital.
- Give the prescribed antibiotics.
  (a)  Intensive drops, e.g. G. chloramphenicol, G. Gentamicin, G. penicillin half-hourly. The frequency will be reduced according to the response.
  (b)  Ointment, e.g. Oc. chloramphenicol and gentamicin at night.
  (c)  Subconjunctival antibiotics.
  (d)  Oral antibiotics may be given.
  (e)  If very severe, intravenous antibiotics may be given.
- Give analgesic drugs as prescribed.
- Give topical mydriatics for associated uveitis.
- If the patient is to be treated as an outpatient, instruct him in the instillation of drops and ointment as above. The frequency may be less, e.g. 2-hourly. Ensure he has analgesics at home.
- Advise him to wear dark glasses for the photophobia and not to cover the eye with a pad.

- Warn him that treatment may be prolonged for several weeks until healing is complete.
- Steroids may be introduced once the ulcer begins to heal.
- Prepare the patient for botulinum injection to induce a ptosis which will cover the cornea.

## Complications

- Scarring of the cornea occurs if the ulcer spreads beyond the epithelial layer.
- Uveitis with its own complications (see Section 9.5.2).
- Descemetocele formation. The elastic Descemet's membrane affords some protection against the spreading ulcer. The corneal layers above it have been destroyed and Descemet's membrane herniates through the ulcer. When this happens perforation may occur.
- Perforation of the cornea. This may be a dangerous situation as not only can sight be lost but the eye itself. If the infection is severe and has spread to the internal structures of the eye, the eye will need to be removed (see Chapter 15), as no useful vision will be saved and the patient will experience severe pain.

### 8.5.3   Corneal ulcers associated with viral infections

### Adenovirus

These cause superficial punctate keratitis – slightly raised dots on the cornea which show up when stained with G. fluorescein. These conditions have been discussed under viral conjunctivitis (see Section 7.2.1).

### Herpes simplex

The herpes simplex virus causes an ulcer on the cornea which has a typical branching pattern and is called a 'dendritic ulcer'. It is usually unilateral.

### *Signs*

- Red eye.
- Dendritic ulcer (Fig. 8.3) seen on the cornea once stained with G. fluorescein.
- Herpes simplex lesions may be evident around the eye.
- Cold sores may be present around the mouth and/or nose.

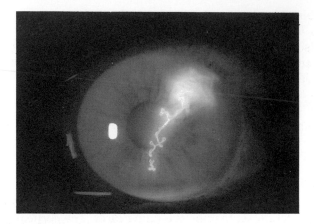

**Fig. 8.3** Dendritic ulcer from herpes simplex virus.

*Patient's needs*

• Relief of symptoms:
 (a) irritation;
 (b) watering;
 (c) photophobia;
 (d) reduced vision.
Pain may not be a symptom as the cornea may have become anaesthetised by the virus.
• Treatment for the infection.

*Nursing action*

• Take swabs for herpes simplex virus isolation.
• Instruct the patient on the treatment with antiviral agents: Oc. aciclovir 5 times a day.
  Treatment is given for a week initially but may need to be continued for longer.
• Steroids are *never* used for herpes simplex infection because they increase the activity of the virus and the possibility of secondary infection. Perforation of the cornea has been caused by the use of steroids.
• Aciclovir cream can be applied to affected skin areas.

*Complications*

• *Amoeboid or geographical ulcer.* The dendritic ulcer spreads to take on the appearance of an amoeba or island.
• *Disciform keratitis.* The stromal layer becomes oedematous and there

are folds in Descemet's membrane. The complaint occurs in patients who are immunosuppressed. It is usually a self-limiting condition lasting several weeks, but may become chronic, in which case uveitis also occurs. A very low dose of steroids may then be required. Prednisolone sodium phosphate can then be produced in a weak solution such as 0.003%.

* Corneal scarring from repeated attacks of herpes simplex keratitis.

    If a corneal graft is performed, the herpes virus can attack the grafted cornea.

### Herpes zoster ophthalmicus

This is caused by the herpes zoster virus attacking the ophthalmic division of the trigeminal nerve (Fig. 8.4). It therefore follows the path of the nerve over the forehead and into the eye. It usually affects the elderly and can be very debilitating. The disease starts with pain over the forehead and scalp on the affected side. A day or so later vesicles appear on the same area and may cover the upper lid. These then break down and weep serous fluid before drying up and forming scabs. The patient feels ill, anorexic and nauseated and may be pyrexial.

    If the nasociliary nerve is affected, the cornea will be involved with white infiltrate and lesions may appear on the side of the nose.

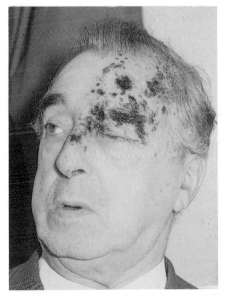

**Fig. 8.4** Herpes zoster ophthalmicus.

*Patient's needs* (see Advice Sheet No. 4)

- Relief of symptoms, especially pain.
- Admission to hospital if the condition is severe or if the patient is elderly and cannot manage at home.
- Institution of treatment.

*Nursing action*

Ensure the patient understands the treatment.
  (a) Skin lesions:
      (i)   aciclovir cream can be applied twice a day to the vesicles;
      (ii)  hydrocortisone cream can also be used.

---

**ADVICE SHEET No. 4**
**Eye Casualty Department**

# SHINGLES
# (Herpes zoster)

Shingles (herpes zoster) is caused by the chicken pox virus. This virus can stay hidden and inactive in anyone who has had chicken pox and then years later, can become active again, producing shingles. It causes a painful rash which affects one side of the face and scalp. If the eye itself becomes involved the vision may become blurred or the eye may become red and sore.

The treatment of shingles is with tablets and cream to the skin. If the eye is involved you will have eye ointment. You must take this as prescribed by the doctor.

It is advisable to have your own towel and flannel while the rash lasts because shingles is infectious (you can give people chicken pox).

Shingles can be a very painful and debilitating condition and the skin may be sensitive to touch. Your own GP will be able to provide strong painkillers and sometimes sleeping tablets if you need them. The rash may take several weeks to completely disappear.

**Further advice & instructions**

. . . . . . . . . . . . . . . . . . . . . . . . . . . . . . . . . . . . . . . . . . . . . . . . . . . . . . . . . . . . . . . . . . . . . .

. . . . . . . . . . . . . . . . . . . . . . . . . . . . . . . . . . . . . . . . . . . . . . . . . . . . . . . . . . . . . . . . . . . . . .

. . . . . . . . . . . . . . . . . . . . . . . . . . . . . . . . . . . . . . . . . . . . . . . . . . . . . . . . . . . . . . . . . . . . . .

. . . . . . . . . . . . . . . . . . . . . . . . . . . . . . . . . . . . . . . . . . . . . . . . . . . . . . . . . . . . . . . . . . . . . .

    (b)   Corneal involvement:

        (i)    antiviral agents, e.g. Oc. aciclovir 5 times a day. Aciclovir can also be given orally;

        (ii)   antibiotics, e.g. G. chloramphenicol 4 times a day to prevent a superimposed bacterial infection;

        (iii)  steroids, e.g. betamethasone sodium phosphate drops 4 times a day, and a mydriatic, e.g. homatropine 2% twice a day, to prevent or treat uveitis.

    (c)   Pain: oral analgesics such as paracetamol given regularly 4-hourly. Stronger analgesics such as mefenamic acid or dextropropoxyphene may be necessary.

        Anti-inflammatory and anti-epileptic agents have been tried to treat the pain. Night sedation or an antidepressant at night may be required.

    (d)   Advise the patient that he will feel unwell and will require a light diet and plenty of fluids.

        Warn the patient that although the unaffected eyelid may swell in apparent sympathy, it will not be affected by the virus.

### Complications

50% of patients develop ocular complications.

(a)   Uveitis.
(b)   Glaucoma.
(c)   Cataract.
(d)   Conjunctivitis.
(e)   Keratitis.
(f)   Permanent corneal scarring.
(g)   Anaesthetic cornea due to the nasociliary nerve being damaged by the virus. The cornea is then exposed to damage because the corneal reflex is absent. Bandage contact lenses or protective arms on spectacles can be worn. This may resolve over months or years.
(h)   More rarely, optic neuritis; scleritis; paralysis of the third, fourth and sixth cranial nerves.
(i)   Partial ptosis due to scarring of lid from vesicles.
(j)   Post-herpetic neuralgia is the most debilitating complication which can last intermittently for several years following the initial attack. It is difficult to treat and may require attendance at a pain clinic.

These complications can occur 6–10 years after the initial attack.

### 8.5.4   Interstitial keratitis

Interstitial keratitis is due to congenital syphilis, manifesting itself when the patient is aged between 5 and 20 years. The patient complains of pain, watering eye, photophobia and blepharospasm and reduced vision. The eye is red and the cornea oedematous. Other signs of congenital syphilis may be present: saddle nose, deafness and notched incisor teeth.

There is no specific treatment. Any treatment given is aimed at preventing uveitis and the formation of posterior synechiae by giving mydriatics and steroid drops. Wearing dark glasses may help the photophobia. Corneal grafting may be necessary if corneal scarring becomes severe enough to obscure vision.

### 8.5.5  Bullous keratopathy

Bullous keratopathy is prolonged oedema of the cornea resulting in the epithelium being raised into large vesicles or bullae. It is a difficult condition to treat and the bullae may burst periodically causing intense irritating symptoms. It occurs following disturbance to the endothelium when aqueous is allowed to percolate into the stroma. This could be as a result of trauma, surgery (especially intra-ocular lens implants) or long-standing, poorly controlled glaucoma.

Hypertonic saline drops can be used. Grafting may be necessary. The excimer laser may be employed (Thomann *et al.* 1985). Bandage contact lenses make the condition less painful.

### 8.5.6  Corneal dystrophies

Corneal dystrophies can be categorised according to the corneal layer involved:

- *epithelial/anterior*  Gogan's, map–dot, recurrent erosions, Reis–Bückler;
- *stromal*  granular, macular, lattice;
- *endothelial/posterior*  Fuchs'.

These dystrophies cause increasing visual loss. Corneal grafting is the main form of treatment but the dystrophy can recur in the 'new' cornea. Recurrent erosions can be treated with the excimer laser.

### 8.5.7  Keratoconus

Keratoconus or conical cornea is due to a congenital weakness of the cornea, manifesting itself in the early teens. It can be associated with conditions such as eczema, mental retardation or blindness as sufferers of these conditions tend to rub their eyes.

It is a bilateral condition, one eye usually being affected before the other. The central cornea becomes progressively thinner and more conical in shape (Fig. 8.5). The patient complains of blurred vision due to increasing astigmatism of the cornea.

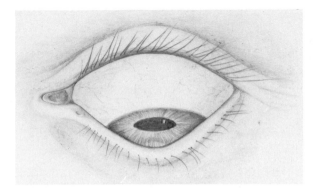

**Fig. 8.5** Keratoconus. (Reproduced with permission from Miller, S. *Parson's Diseases of the Eye*, 16th edn, Churchill Livingstone.)

### Signs

- Munson's sign (see Fig. 8.5). When the patient looks downwards, the conical cornea causes an indentation of the lower lid margin.
- Distorted corneal reflection with Placido's Disc, a keratoscope, a pachometer or ISIS machine.
- An irregular shadow on retinoscopy.
- Unclear view of fundus because of the corneal distortion.

### Treatment

Initially the treatment will be with contact lenses to correct the astigmatism and protect the cornea. The astigmatism is too severe to be corrected by spectacles. As the conical shape progresses, an ordinary contact lens becomes of no use. Grafting is performed, ideally before the cornea becomes too thin

### Complications

- Perforation of the cornea.

### 8.5.8 Keratoplasty – corneal graft

Keratoplasty needs to be performed when the cornea is so diseased that the patient's vision is lost (Fig. 8.6). It is performed for (in order of occurrence):

(a) keratoconus;
(b) bullous keratopathy;
(c) scarring/injury;

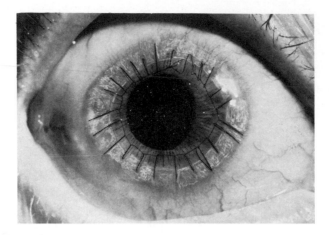

**Fig. 8.6** Corneal graft.

(d)   corneal dystrophies;
(e)   corneal ulcers;
(f)   dendritic ulcers;
(g)   failed previous grafts.

### 8.5.9   Eye donors

- *Autogenous.* Rarely, a patient requiring a corneal graft has a fellow eye which is blind but with a healthy cornea which can be used for grafting.
- *Live donor.* An enucleated eye with a healthy cornea can be used for grafting onto another patient.
- *Cadavers.* Most of the corneas used for grafting are obtained by this method. They must be removed within 12 hours of death and are stored in media. Organ culture medium permits storage for up to 30 days.
    Donor corneas are not used from the following categories:
    (a)   corneal disease;
    (b)   anterior segment surgery or disease;
    (c)   HIV or hepatitis B positive and drug abuse;
    (d)   death of unknown cause;
    (e)   septicaemia;
    (f)   leukaemia, Hodgkin's disease, lymphosarcoma.
    A culture is taken from the eyes before removal to exclude any infection. Blood is taken to exclude hepatitis B and HIV. Both eyes are taken, including a part of the optic nerve. A suture is fed through the nerve and used to suspend the eye in a sterile jar to prevent the cornea becoming damaged. A prosthesis might be put in each socket or the eyelids are sutured together.

There is a national Eye Donor Bank in Bristol (UK) which stores eyes waiting for recipients.

### 8.5.10   Eye recipients

*Patient's needs*

- Admission to hospital
- Pre-and post-operative care.

*Nursing action*

- The nurse needs to ascertain that the patient understands that he will be receiving a donor cornea which is most likely to come from a cadaver. The use of the word 'graft' instead of 'transplant' may result in the patient being unaware of the true implications of this type of surgery. The nurse may want to involve the doctor or may discuss this with the patient on her own. Some patients may be distressed at the knowledge. Others having known for a while, may only face up to the fact at the time of surgery, while some may not have had the opportunity for discussion before. The nurse needs to be aware of those who require further discussion and talk it through with them.
  Admit the patient to the ward.
- Institute pre-operative care. The pupil is constricted to prevent damage to the lens during the operation unless a cataract is to be removed at the same time.
- Carry out post-operative care. At the first dressing ensure that the graft is in place, the sutures intact and that the anterior chamber is formed. Aqueous may have leaked through the suture line causing a flat anterior chamber. Instil antibiotic or antibiotic and steroid and mydriatic drops.
- Patients need to be advised about the signs of rejection: reduced vision, red eye, new vessel growth around the cornea and pain.

Following corneal grafting astigmatism may occur which will require correction by the wearing of spectacles or contact lenses.

*Complications*

*Short term*

- Damage during the operation to the iris or lens.
- Aqueous leak from the graft which has lifted in one area. This will require resuturing.

- Infection requiring antibiotics.

*Long term*

- Neovascularisation around the edge of the graft. No treatment is required unless vision is impaired. Beta rays can be used on the area to destroy the new blood vessels. Regrafting may be necessary.
- Astigmatism caused by too tight sutures which may need adjusting. Topography can confirm this.
- Warping of donor graft caused by sutures that are too loose. This may require resuturing.
- Rejection which will be treated with steroids. Compared with other transplant operations, keratoplasty does not present the same rejection problems as the cornea does not have a blood supply.

## 8.6 CONDITIONS AFFECTING THE SCLERA

### 8.6.1 Scleritis

Scleritis is a rare condition affecting women more than men. In 50% of cases it is associated with connective tissue diseases, such as rheumatoid arthritis and ankylosing spondylitis. It can also be associated with uveitis, glaucoma and cataract. If it is anterior, the eye will be red, with tenderness over the affected area. If it is posterior, the eye will look white. Pain is the main feature and may be severe. Steroid drops will be used for anterior scleritis and systemic anti-inflammatory drugs such as ibuprofen for posterior scleritis.

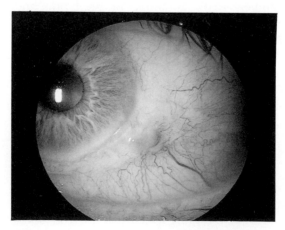

**Fig. 8.7** Episcleritis.

### 8.6.2   Episcleritis

Episcleritis is inflammation of the episclera (Fig. 8.7). It may be unilateral or bilateral and can be associated with rheumatoid arthritis, gout and ulcerative colitis but the cause is often unknown.

There is a localised area of redness, usually triangular, with the apex pointing towards the limbus. There may or may not be a nodule present in the area of redness. The area is tender and, on examination, the conjunctiva moves freely over the enlarged episcleral blood vessels. Treatment is with steroid drops such as prednisolone sodium phosphate.

# 9 The Uveal Tract

## 9.1 INTRODUCTION

The uveal tract comprises the middle vascular pigmented layer of the eye. It is composed of three areas:

(1) the *choroid*, which forms the posterior five-sixths;
(2) the *ciliary body*;
(3) the *iris*.

These two latter structures (Fig. 9.1) together form the anterior one-sixth.

## 9.2 THE CHOROID

The choroid lies between the sclera and retina and extends from the optic nerve forwards to the ora serrata where it joins the ciliary body. It is composed of four layers:

(1) the *suprachoroid*, containing pigment cells, elastic tissue and collagen;
(2) the *vascular layer*, comprising large and small blood vessels with pigment cells contained in the stroma surrounding the vessels. The large vessels are mainly veins;
(3) the *choriocapillaries*, comprising fenestrated capillary vessels;
(4) *Bruch's membrane*, which is a barrier with fenestrations which allow nutrients through to the underlying retina. It is also a supportive membrane.

### 9.2.1 Function of the choroid

The function of the choroid is to provide nourishment to the outer layer of the underlying retina.

### 9.2.2 Blood supply

The blood supply and drainage is via:

- short posterior ciliary artery;
- choroidal and vortex veins.

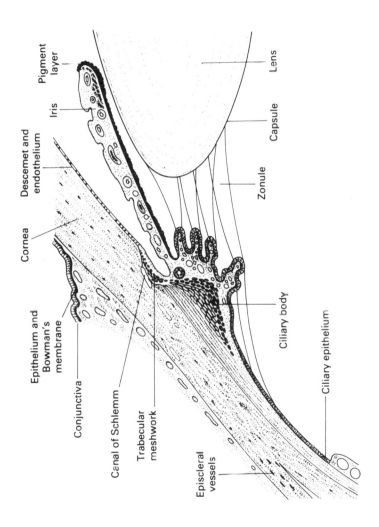

**Fig. 9.1** Section through the iris and ciliary region.

### 9.2.3    Nerve supply

The posterior ciliary nerve from the oculomotor nerve provides the nerve supply to the choroid.

## 9.3    THE CILIARY BODY

The ciliary body is a triangular structure lying between the choroid and the iris, being 6 mm wide.

There are three areas.

(1)  The *pars plana* is the posterior aspect lying next to the ora serrata and is 4 mm wide.
(2)  The *pars plicata* is the area which lies between the pars plana and the iris and is 2 mm wide. It contains 70–80 radiating strips, the *ciliary processes*. These processes are composed of vascular tissue, mainly veins and capillaries. They are 2 mm long and 0.5 mm wide. Their function is to produce and secrete aqueous which fills the posterior chamber, and then flows through the pupil into the anterior chamber. The *zonular fibres* or *suspensory ligaments*, which hold the lens in place, originate in the valleys formed by the processes.
(3)  The *ciliary muscles* lie in the anterior section of the ciliary body, underneath the sclera. The ciliary muscles are known as the *muscles of accommodation*. They contract and relax to change the shape of the lens so that light rays can be brought to a focus on the retina when looking at objects at varying distances. When the ciliary muscles contract, the zonules relax and decrease the tension on the lens capsule. The lens thus becomes more spherical and light rays can be focused on the retina for near vision. When the ciliary muscles relax, the zonules tighten and there is increased tension on the lens capsule. The lens thus becomes less spherical and light rays are focused on the retina for distance vision.

### 9.3.1    Blood supply

The blood supply to and drainage from the ciliary body is via:

• anterior ciliary arteries and veins;
• long posterior ciliary arteries and veins;
• vortex vein.

### 9.3.2    Nerve supply

The nerve supply is through the short ciliary nerve from the oculomotor nerve.

## 9.4 THE IRIS

The iris is the coloured circular diaphragm situated behind the cornea and in front of the lens. It is attached at its periphery to the ciliary body. The pupil is the aperture in the middle of the iris. The iris forms the posterior wall of the anterior chamber and the anterior wall of the posterior chamber.

There are two zones:

(1)  the *ciliary zone* on the periphery;
(2)  the *pupillary zone* on the central aspect.

### 9.4.1  Three layers of the iris

(1)  The *endothelium.*
(2)  The *stroma* containing connective tissue, pigment cells, blood vessels, nerves and muscles.
(3)  *Pigment epithelium* which is an extension of the pigment epithelium of the retina.

Note that the epithelium of the iris is situated at the back of the structure.

### 9.4.2  Muscle of the iris

There are two muscles in the iris, whose actions are either to constrict or dilate the pupil.

(1)  The *sphincter muscle* is a circular muscle lying around the pupillary zone. This muscle constricts the pupil. It is served by the short ciliary nerve of the oculomotor nerve.
(2)  The *dilator muscle* is a radial muscle lying under the pigmented layer of the iris. As its name indicates it is the muscle that dilates the pupil and is supplied by the long ciliary nerve from the nasociliary nerve, the third branch of the ophthalmic division of the trigeminal nerve.

The sphincter muscle is more powerful than the dilator muscle, so if both muscles are equally affected by intra-ocular inflammation the pupil will tend to constrict.

The sphincter muscle and the ciliary muscle both have their nerve supply from the oculomotor nerve, therefore drugs stimulating or paralysing this nerve will affect both dilation and accommodation.

### 9.4.3    Colour of the iris

The pigment melanin gives the colour to the iris. The colour depends on the amount of pigment laid down in the stroma after birth. This is genetically determined. The pigment in the pigment epithelium is present at birth and is consistent throughout life. This gives newborn babies light-coloured eyes. After a few days of life pigment begins to be laid down in the stroma and the baby's eyes become darker. The more melanin laid down, the darker the eyes become. All babies are therefore born with light-coloured eyes, despite what some doting parents may say! The amount of pigment produced in the stroma can vary during life, so that the colour of eyes can alter. Dark irises with dense pigment cause the pupil to take longer to dilate following instillation of mydriatics.

### 9.4.4    Blood supply

The arterial blood supply is via the long posterior ciliary arteries. The capillaries from these arteries anastomose with the anterior ciliary arteries to form the *arterial circle of the iris.*

The venous drainage is through the anterior ciliary veins and vortex veins.

## 9.5    CONDITIONS OF THE UVEAL TRACT

### 9.5.1    Choroiditis

Choroiditis is a condition manifesting itself as patches of inflammation on the choroid. On examination with an ophthalmoscope fluffy white patches can be seen through a hazy vitreous. When these patches heal, they leave pigmented areas of scar tissue.

### Symptoms

The patient complains of reduced vision due to infiltrates in the vitreous and of an increased number of vitreous floaters. In 60% of cases, the cause is unknown. It can be caused by toxocara, toxoplasmosis or syphilis. If the cause is known, this should be treated. A short course of high-dose steroids is also given.

### Complications

* Cataract due to defective nourishment of the lens.
* Optic neuritis and secondary optic atrophy.
* Retinal changes and progressive degeneration, resulting in retinal atrophy. A decrease in the size of the visual field will be noted.

### 9.5.2 Anterior uveitis or iritis (Fig. 9.2)

Anterior uveitis or iritis is inflammation of the iris or iris and ciliary body. It is usually a recurring condition in which the cause is unknown in 70% of cases.

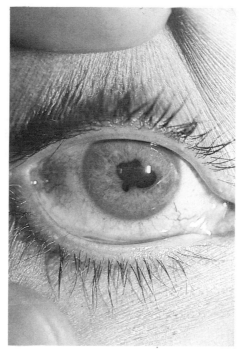

**Fig. 9.2** Acute iritis.

### Causes

Causes of anterior uveitis, in order of occurrence, are:

(1) ankylosing spondylitis;
(2) Still's disease or childhood arthritis;
(3) seronegative rheumatoid disease;
(4) ophthalmic surgery;
(5) trauma – perforating injury, corneal foreign body;
(6) corneal ulcer;
(7) sarcoid;
(8) tuberculosis;
(9) syphilis;
(10) ulcerative colitis and Crohn's disease;
(11) rarely, neovascularisation from diabetes mellitus;

(12)  also rarely, heterochromic uveitis. Patients with different coloured irises may develop this chronic, progressive condition in which the pigment of the affected eye is dislodged, with the iris becoming gradually paler.

## Signs

- Limbal injection.
- Cornea is usually clear. Keratic precipitates may be present on the posterior surface of the cornea if the inflammation is severe. These are plaques of precipitates from the inflamed iris. In tuberculosis or sarcoid these are particularly marked and are called 'mutton fat' because of their appearance.
- The anterior chamber is of normal depth but 'flare and cells' may be seen in the beam of the slit lamp. These are the albumin exudates from the inflamed iris floating in the anterior chamber. These cells may be sufficient in number to settle and form a hypopyon.
- The iris is swollen and looks 'muddy'. A nodule may be present if the cause is tuberculosis.
- The intra-ocular pressure may be initially low if the ciliary processes are involved because they will produce less aqueous. The pressure is never raised unless secondary glaucoma has occurred.
- The pupil is small because the iris muscles are in spasm and the sphincter muscle is the stronger of the two iris muscles. The pupil will be irregular if posterior synaechiae has occurred when the posterior surface of the swollen iris adheres to the anterior surface of the lens.

## Patient's needs (see Advice Sheet No. 5)

- Relief of symptoms:
    (a)  pain due to the spasm of the nerves of the iris;
    (b)  photophobia ⎱ due to irritation of the nerves
    (c)  watering eye ⎰ of the iris;
    (d)  reduced visual acuity due to the presence of flare and cells in the anterior chamber.
- Investigation of the cause in recurrent cases, and treatment, if applicable.
- Institution of treatment.

## Nursing action

- Dilation of the pupil to prevent posterior synaechiae from forming or to break down any that have formed.
    (a)  Instil prescribed mydriatic drops, often a 'cocktail' will be used, e.g. G. homatropine 2%, G. phenylephrine hydrochloride 10% and

---

**ADVICE SHEET No. 5**
**Eye Casualty Department**

# IRITIS

**What is iritis?**

The iris is the coloured part of your eye, and iritis simply means that this has become inflamed. This usually causes misty vision, redness of the eye and a dull ache which is worse in bright light.

**Why have I got iritis?**

In many people the cause of iritis is unknown, sometimes people get iritis in association with other conditions outside the eye and a lot of research is being done into this. You will probably have some tests done to see if there is any associated general health condition.

**How Is iritis treated?**

Most people with iritis respond to eye drops within a few days. The drops used are:

(1) **Steroids**. These are given throughout the day as eye drops (such as Maxidex, or Predsol) and at night as a longer acting cream (e.g. Betnesol). As your symptoms improve your doctor will suggest that you gradually reduce the number of drops you use each day.

(2) **Drops to dilate the pupil**. e.g. atropine or cyclopentolate. These make the vision blurred and can interfere with driving. They are necessary in the early stages of an attack and make the eye feel more comfortable and avoid damaging complications.

**Will the iritis come back again?**

Not infrequently, iritis tends to recur and it is important that you go to an eye unit if your symptoms return, so that you can be treated promptly.

---

G. cyclopentolate 1%. These may need to be repeated if synaechiae are present.

(b) Sykes heater (see Section 3.2.22) will enhance the action of the mydriatics and cause the pupil to dilate quicker. The heat will also afford some pain relief.

(c) A subconjunctival injection of mydriatics, e.g. atropine (Mydricaine) may need to be given (see Section 3.2.14).

• Steroid drops will be instilled. A subconjunctival injection of a steroid, e.g. betamethasone sodium phosphate 4 mg may need to be given in severe cases.

- Ensure the patient understands the treatment to be instilled at home. This will be:
  (a)   a mydriatic, e.g. G. homatropine 2% twice a day;
  (b)   a steroid, e.g. dexamethasone hourly or 2-hourly.
- If investigations are to be carried out, ensure the patient understands where and when to attend for these. These tests will include: X-rays – skull, chest and joints to exclude sarcoid, tuberculosis, arthritis and ankylosing spondylitis; blood tests – haemoglobin, full blood count, erythrocyte sedimentation rate, serology and autoimmune profile.
- Ensure the patient knows when to return for follow-up treatment which will probably be in one or two days' time.

## Complications

- Secondary glaucoma from three causes.
  (a)   Posterior synaechiae, if not broken down, can cause a ring synaechiae when all of the pupillary zone of the iris is bound down to the anterior lens surface. The aqueous cannot flow through the pupil, so as the pressure builds up in the posterior chamber, the iris is pushed forward. This condition is known as iris bombe. Ring synaechiae can be divided surgically if mydriatics do not cause the pupil to dilate and thus break the synaechiae.
  (b)   The peripheral anterior surface of the iris bombe adheres to the peripheral posterior surface of the cornea causing peripheral anterior synaechiae. These block the drainage angle.
  (c)   Debris from the inflamed iris blocks the drainage angle.
- Visual impairment from iris pigment in the pupil.
- Cataract formation from impairment of the metabolism of the lens.
- Hypopyon of sterile pus.
- Cystoid macular oedema (see Section 12.7.3).

### 9.5.3   Tumours

Benign naevi can be present in the uveal tract. They must be observed carefully and regularly for malignant changes. They can be removed by laser. Melanomas are the variety of malignant tumour affecting the uveal tract. They are more common in the choroid, but can occur in the iris and, more rarely, in the ciliary body where they carry a higher mortality.

### Melanoma of the choroid

This can occur at any age but is more common over the age of 55 years. It usually occurs in the posterior pole and as it grows it pushes the retina forwards. A retinal detachment thus caused is often the first sign of a melanoma, so careful differential diagnoses must be made between a malignant and a simple retinal detachment. The edge of a malignant detachment is usually smoother than that of a simple detachment. Investigations include transillumination, colour fundus photography and ocular ultrasound. Treatment is with ruthenium or iodine plaques, proton beam radiotherapy, trans-scleral or trans-vitreal local resection or laser photocoagulation. The aim is to conserve the eye. Enucleation is reserved for patients who have visual loss, pain and poor cosmetic appearance, and those who are unable to cope with the thought of tumour spread or with prolonged treatment and follow-up. A length of optic nerve must also be removed with the whole eyeball. If the optic nerve is found to be involved on histological examination, radiotherapy should be given to the socket. The five-year mortality rate varies from 16% for small tumours less than 10 mm in diameter to 53% for tumours larger than 15 mm (Damato 1995). (For nursing care following enucleation see Section 15.12.)

### Melanoma of the iris

If a naevus in the iris is noted to be enlarging, local excision should be performed. The prognosis, providing treatment is prompt, is usually good.

# 10 Glaucoma

## 10.1 INTRODUCTION

Glaucoma is a rise in the intra-ocular pressure that is sufficient to cause damage to the ocular structures. Intra-ocular pressure is determined by the balance between the rate of production and the rate of drainage of aqueous fluid. Normal intra-ocular pressure is 15–20 mmHg, but this measurement depends to some extent on which method is used to measure it.

## 10.2 METHODS OF MEASURING INTRA-OCULAR PRESSURE

### 10.2.1 Digital

The patient looks downwards, closing the eye to be examined, and the nurse gently palpates the eyeball to assess the degree of 'hardness'. No accurate measurement can be taken but an eye with raised pressure will feel harder than one with normal pressure. It is a useful initial method of assessment, especially if none of the specialised equipment needed for measuring intra-ocular pressure is available, as in the GP's surgery.

### 10.2.2 Goldmann applanation tonometer

The tonometer head is attached to a slit lamp. The eye is anaesthetised with anaesthetic drops and fluorescein drops are also instilled. The tonometer head is placed against the cornea and the pressure measurement is read off a dial on the tonometer. Normal pressure is 10–20 mmHg (see Section 3.2.25).

### 10.2.3 Perkins' applanation tonometer

The Perkins' applanation tonometer is a hand-held tonometer, working on the principles of the Goldmann tonometer mentioned above. It is useful for patients who are unable to sit at a slit lamp, e.g. those who are in wheelchairs, who are bedbound or unconscious. The method of use and normal pressure are the same as for the Goldmann tonometer.

### 10.2.4 Tonopen

Tonopens are small pen-like instruments that measure pressure in a similar fashion to the applanation method.

### 10.2.5 Non-contact tonometer

Non-contract tonometers, employed by optometrists, use a puff of air blown against the eye. The time required to flatten the cornea is converted into a figure to denote the intra-ocular pressure.

## 10.3 THE ANTERIOR CHAMBER

The anterior chamber is the area between the posterior surface of the cornea and the anterior surface of the iris. The angle of the anterior chamber may be examined using a gonioscope (see Section 10.7.1).

## 10.4 THE POSTERIOR CHAMBER

The posterior chamber is the area between the posterior surface of the iris and the anterior surface of the lens and suspensory ligaments. Both these chambers are filled with aqueous fluid.

## 10.5 AQUEOUS FLUID

Aqueous is a clear fluid produced by the ciliary processes of the ciliary body (see Section 9.3). It flows from the ciliary body into the posterior chamber, through the pupil, into the anterior chamber, and drains through the anterior chamber angle at the rate of approximately 2 µl/minute.

### 10.5.1 Composition of aqueous

Aqueous is similar in constitution to plasma: 99% water and 1% nutrients, e.g. sodium, potassium, chloride, bicarbonate.
Volume is approximately 125 µl.

### 10.5.2    Functions of aqueous

- To maintain intra-ocular pressure.
- To provide a clear medium for refraction.
- To provide nourishment to:
  (a)   the lens;
  (b)   the posterior surface of the cornea.

## 10.6    THE ANGLE OF THE ANTERIOR CHAMBER

The angle of the anterior chamber lies between the limbus (corneal–scleral junction) and the iris and it surrounds the circumference of the anterior chamber. It is composed of the trabecular meshwork and the canal of Schlemm (see Fig. 9.1). The trabecular meshwork is made up of fibrous tissue, perforated with oval holes and covered with endothelium, which is continuous with that of the posterior surface of the cornea.

Aqueous drains through these holes from the anterior chamber into the canal of Schlemm. This is an oval-shaped channel lined with endothelium. Collector channels, 25–30, leave the canal of Schlemm and anastomose to form the intrascleral plexus. From here the aqueous drains into the aqueous veins, the vortex veins and the inferior ophthalmic vein. A small percentage of aqueous exits the eye through the veins of the posterior segment of the eye.

### 10.6.1    Function of the angle

The angle is for the drainage of aqueous fluid from the eye into the venous circulation.

### 10.6.2    Blood supply

The blood supply to and drainage from the angle of the anterior chamber is via:

- anterior ciliary arteries;
- aqueous veins.

## 10.7    RELATED DISORDERS – GLAUCOMA

Glaucoma is a rise in the intra-ocular pressure that causes damage to the eye.

The four types of glaucoma, each with a different aetiology, are:

(1)   primary acute glaucoma (PAG);
(2)   chronic open-angle glaucoma (COAG);

(3)  secondary;
(4)  buphthalmos/childhood (ox-eye).

### 10.7.1  Primary acute glaucoma (Acute closed-angle glaucoma)

Primary acute glaucoma (PAG) affects 1 in 1000 over the age of 40. The incidence increases with age and affects women four times more frequently than men.

The condition can be divided into two types:

(1)  primary pupil block;
(2)  primary irido-trabecular block.

### Pupil block

Some 94% of PAG cases are of the pupil block type. The eye which is predisposed to this type has:

- a dome iris;
- an iris that is characteristically bowed forward;
- hypermetropia;
- a shallow anterior chamber;
- a narrow drainage angle;
- a large anteriorly placed lens.

The pupil becomes blocked by the lens when the pupil is semi-dilated. The aqueous cannot flow through the pupil, resulting in a rise in pressure behind the iris. This causes the iris to be pushed forward (iris bombé) and the forward-placed iris blocks the drainage angle. Treatment for this involves the use of miotic drops which brings the iris away from the angle and laser iridotomy which will allow the aqueous to pass into the anterior chamber, bypassing the blocked pupil.

### Irido-trabecular block

Irido-trabecular block only occurs in 6% of PAG cases. In irido-trabecular block the eye typically has:

- a plateau iris;
- emmetropia;
- a deep anterior chamber;
- deeply recessed angles.

Pupillary dilation leads to a progressive irido-trabecular blockage. Treatment is by the use of miotic drops to bring the iris away from the angle.

PAG usually presents unilaterally, but the fellow eye can also be affected, so it must receive prophylactic treatment.

PAG can be divided into five stages which may overlap but the overlap may not be orderly from one stage to the next:

- latent – asymptomatic;
- intermittent or sub-acute;
- acute;
- chronic;
- absolute – end stage.

### Latent

As the patients are asymptomatic the condition is diagnosed either at a routine eye examination or when another eye condition is being investigated. These patients must be warned of the prodromal symptoms (see below) in case they progress to the next stage.

### Intermittent or sub-acute

A rapid closure of parts of the angle (see Gonioscopy below) causes the pressure to rise. This results in certain prodromal symptoms and signs:

- headache;
- eye pain;
- blurred vision      } due to corneal
- haloes seen around lights } oedema;
- nausea.

These prodromal symptoms and signs usually occur at night and improve by the morning when the miosed pupil during sleep has come away from the angle. Patients often think they have a migraine or 'sick headache'. An attack may develop into an acute attack or bypass this stage. As more of the angle becomes blocked with subsequent attacks, chronic closed-angle glaucoma develops. It is therefore important to diagnose and treat this stage early. Treatment is by laser iridotomy followed by intensive miotic drops.

### *Investigations*

#### *Provocative tests*

Provocative tests are performed in patients with prodromal or latent symptoms to see if the intra-ocular pressure rises when the eye has been subjected to certain situations.

- *Dark room test.* The intra-ocular pressure is measured. The patient is then asked to lie prone in a dark room for 1 hour, he must not close his eyes as the pupil will naturally constrict. The prone position is used to see if gravity on the lens causes the angle to narrow even more. After 1 hour, the intra-ocular pressure is taken again. If there has been a rise of 8 mmHg or more the potential for an attack of acute glaucoma to occur is present.
- *Mydriatic test.* The intra-ocular pressure is measured. G. cyclopentolate 1% is instilled to dilate the pupil. The intra-ocular pressure is measured every 15 minutes for 1 hour. Again if there is a rise of over 8 mmHg the potential for an attack of acute glaucoma to occur is present. The effect of the cyclopentolate must be reversed immediately the test has been completed by instilling G. pilocarpine 2–4% intensively until the pupil has returned to normal size, to prevent an acute attack occurring.

*Non-provocative tests*

- *Gonioscopy.* The depth of the patient's anterior chamber angle can be assessed by the use of a gonioscope. This is a large contact lens with either two or three mirrors placed at differing angles to each other (Fig. 10.1). This enables the angle of the anterior chamber to be viewed when used with the slit lamp. The patient's eye is anaesthetised with anaesthetic drops and a lubricant such as methylcellulose is applied to the surface of the lens that is placed against the cornea. This lubricates the lens and fills the space between the lens and the cornea. The degree to which the angle is open is graded from 0 to 4; 0 being closed and 4

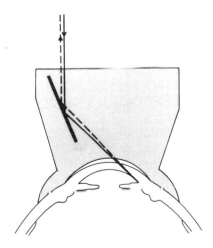

**Fig. 10.1** Optical systems of Goldmann contact lens used in gonioscopy.

being fully open. Grades 1 and 2 demonstrate that angle closure is probable/possible. The circumference of the angle usually has variable degrees of closure.

## Acute

This is an ophthalmic emergency as the pressure can damage the optic nerve irreversibly.

### Signs

A sudden rise in intra-ocular pressure due either to pupil block or angle closure causes congestion and oedema of the structures involved.

- Lids may be red and swollen.
- Conjunctiva may show dusky red injection and may be chemosed.
- Hazy cornea.
- Iris may appear 'muddy' and swollen with loss of its usual clear pattern.
- Pupil may be fixed, semi-dilated and oval in shape.
- Shallow anterior chamber.
- Raised intra-ocular pressure. (Can be as high as 70 mmHg.)
- Rapidly reduced visual acuity.

### Patient's needs

- Relief of symptoms:
  - (a)   severe headache;
  - (b)   pain in the eye;
  - (c)   nausea;
  - (d)   vomiting;
  - (e)   abdominal pain;
  - (f)   generally feeling unwell.

  These symptoms can sometimes be confused with other conditions such as acute abdomen and, with the dilated pupil, neurological conditions.
- Reassurance and explanation.
- Possible admission to hospital.
- Preparation for laser treatment.
- Instructions on discharge from hospital.

### Nursing priorities

- Inform medical staff at once. Immediate treatment will bring relief of symptoms and prevent complications occurring.

- Prepare medication and commence instillation of drops as soon as possible after they have been prescribed.

*Immediate nursing action*

Test visual acuity, if patient is fit enough.

- Explain that treatment to the eye will relieve general symptoms.
- Lay the patient on a couch in a quiet, darkened area.
- Give the patient a vomit bowl.
- He may appreciate a cold compress on the forehead.
- Prepare acetazolamide 500 mg to be given intravenously by the doctor to reduce the production of aqueous.
- Commence the instillation of G. pilocarpine 4% to the affected eye once it has been prescribed. Intensive miotics are not effective in pulling away the iris from the angle as the sphincter muscle is usually ischaemic if the pressure is above 30 mmHg (Kanski 1994).
- Commence G. pilocarpine 1–2% times a day to unaffected eye.
- Commence a beta-blocker (e.g. Betagan – levobunolol hydrochloride) to the affected eye.
- Commence a steroid drop to the affected eye as there is usually an associated inflammation.
- Give analgesics and/or anti-emetics if headache and nausea and vomiting continue despite treatment.
- Prepare further treatment if necessary to reduce the intra-ocular pressure if initial treatment has failed to bring it down:
  (a) intravenous mannitol 20%–200 ml given over 1–2 hours:
      (i) care for intravenous rate of flow and the site of the cannula, as leakage into the surrounding tissues causes phlebitis;
      (ii) assist the patient to the toilet or give a urinal or bedpan as mannitol has a diuretic effect;
  (b) glycerol (1–5 mg/kg body weight) orally, in orange juice to disguise the taste. This in itself may induce nausea and vomiting.

The patient may resent the frequent attention he requires in the initial stages of treatment of this condition and may just want to be left alone. Handle the patient sympathetically and show understanding of his feelings.

*Further nursing action*

- Prepare the patient for laser iridotomy to both eyes (prophylactically to the fellow eye) if the cause is pupil block.

## Chronic

Often referred to as 'creeping angle closure', this is when repeated attacks of either intermittent or untreated acute episodes cause further adhesions of the peripheral iris to the posterior surface of the cornea (peripheral anterior synechiae), thus closing the angle. The signs and symptoms are similar to chronic *open*-angle glaucoma (see Section 10.7.2).

## Absolute

This is the end stage of primary acute, chronic and secondary (see Sections 10.7.2 and 10.7.3) glaucoma when treatment has failed. Cataracts occur due to the medical or surgical treatment rather than to the disease process (Kuppens *et al.* 1995).

Blind, painful eyes which occur at this stage are best treated by enucleation (see Chapter 15). Alternatively, periodic retrobulbar or facial nerve injections can be administered. Phthisis bulbi, or shrinkage of the eye, occurs as it atrophies when enucleation is the most appropriate course of action.

### 10.7.2    Chronic open-angle glaucoma

Chronic open-angle glaucoma occurs in patients of either sex over the age of 45 years with symptoms occurring after the age of 65 if the disease is undetected. This is not to be confused with the chronic form of primary acute glaucoma. It has an insidious onset and is slowly progressive. Symptoms are not usually noticed by the patient until the disease has progressed so far as to result in marked visual loss. It is a bilateral condition, one eye often being involved earlier and more severely than the other. The patient usually first notices that he cannot see so well in his peripheral vision and has started knocking into things. He often thinks it is just old age or something a new pair of glasses will correct. Hence these patients are often referred to ophthalmologists by opticians.

### Cause

The cause of chronic glaucoma is not really understood, but there are several risk factors (Kanski 1994):

- high myopia;
- central retinal vein occlusion;
- retinal detachment caused by a retinal hole;
- Fuchs' dystrophy;
- increasing age;
- diabetes mellitus;
- raised systolic blood pressure.

There is also a higher incidence in the Afro-Caribbean population (Laske *et al.* 1994).

The aqueous cannot drain away and the intra-ocular pressure rises. The optic nerve head is composed of millions of nerve fibres as they exit the eye. Where the central retinal artery and vein enter and exit through the middle of these fibres, this is referred to as the optic cup. In open-angle glaucoma the cup becomes larger as the nerve fibres atrophy, due to the pressure on them, producing loss of peripheral vision. Typically there is a loss in the nasal peripheral field at first, with progressive loss of the rest of the peripheral field (Fig. 10.2). Central vision is usually retained longer, but will also be lost if treatment is not given or is unsuccessful. Sometimes patients experience loss of central vision before peripheral vision has been affected.

Chronic glaucoma affects 2% of the population and is familial in 10% of cases (Kanski 1994). Anyone with relatives with this disease should receive an ophthalmic check-up, which is free, every 3–5 years after the age of 50 years. Treatment can then be given as soon as signs occur, before symptoms are noted, so that sight can be saved.

## Investigations

Perimetry, ophthalmoscopy and tonometry are carried out to diagnose and monitor the disease.

### Perimetry (see Section 3.2.28)

These tests are performed to assess the degree of peripheral and central visual loss. They are used to detect the disease and follow its progress.

There are several different types of test but they all use the same principle. The patient, with one eye covered, stares at a white spot or light. Without moving his eye from this spot or light he indicates verbally or by pressing a buzzer as soon as he sees another spot or light entering his peripheral vision from any angle in the 360° circle. Most machines these days are computerised.

### Ophthalmoscopy

Examination of the optic disc can be made using an ophthalmoscope to assess the degree of cupping.

### Laser scanning tomography

This is a more sophisticated investigation of the optic disc which quantifies the areas of neural tissue at the optic disc by taking sections through the nerve head in a similar manner to a CT scan.

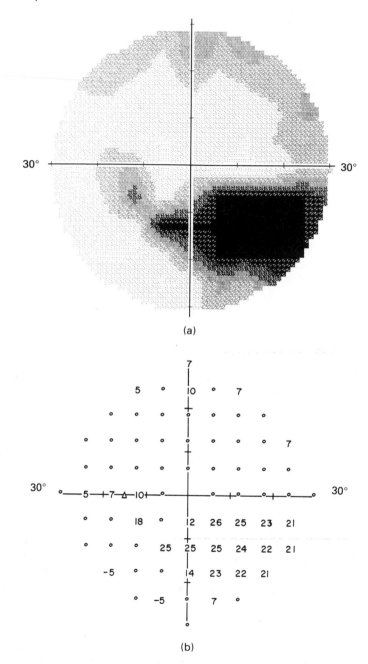

(a)

(b)

**Fig. 10.2** Automated perimeter showing field loss which is shown as (a) a dark grey scale or (b) as high figures or (c) as low figures.

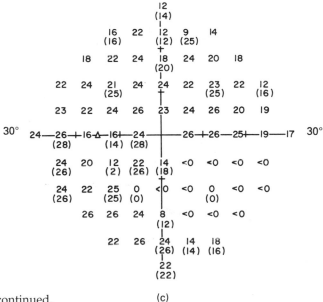

**Fig. 10.2** continued.                    (c)

*Tonometry* (see Section 3.2.25)

Measurement of the intra-ocular pressure is recorded. The pressure is not always markedly raised, especially early in the disease.

*Gonioscopy*

Gonioscopy will be carried out to assess the degree to which the angle is open (see Section 10.3). Patients may have narrow angles as well as chronic glaucoma.

*Phasing*

The patient may be admitted to hospital or attend as a day case to see if the intra-ocular pressure is raised at various times of the day. There is a normal diurnal pattern with the pressure being higher in the mornings. The intra-ocular pressure must be recorded every 4–6 hours, ideally by the same operator.

**Signs**

• Cupped optic disc. The disc becomes oval vertically, and pale with the blood vessels being displaced nasally and the nerve fibre rim becoming narrower. A normal cup is 0.3; a glaucomatous cup is 0.5–0.8. (These values are expressed as ratios – the diameter of the cup is expressed as a fraction of the diameter of the disc giving a cup:disc ratio.)

- Loss of visual fields, typically peripheral field initially and central field later (Fig. 10.2).
- Raised intra-ocular pressure up to 25 mmHg.

## Patient's needs

- Guidance/help with mobility because of visual impairment.
- Assistance with investigations, especially perimetry.
- Instruction in instillation of drops and taking of tablets and disease process and treatment options.
- Preparation for laser treatment or surgery.

## Nursing action

- Guide/help patient while he is in the hospital. He will have varying degrees of visual impairment. If he has peripheral field loss, he will tend to knock into furniture, doors, etc., and will need to be escorted to the varying departments of the hospital he will be attending on a hospital visit.
- Assist the patient with or perform perimetry. These tests require concentration on the part of the patient who tends to be elderly so this is not easy to maintain and therefore the patient needs encouragement and assistance during these tests.
- Give the patient information on his treatment option which will be either:
  - (a)  medical – it is not wise to employ more than two topical medications as changes to the conjunctiva which may occur after three years' use may compromise the success of a trabeculectomy (Broadway *et al.* 1994).
  - (b)  laser – effective in short-term control (Migdal 1995).
  - (c)  surgical – (see Patient Information Leaflet No. 3) surgery is now being performed earlier in the disease than in the past (Migdal 1994). When performed early in the disease the intra-ocular pressure is well controlled (Migdal 1995). It is important to emphasise that lost sight cannot be restored and that the aim of treatment is to preserve what sight is remaining.

## *Medical treatment*

- As compliance can be a particular problem in this condition (Williams 1993; Patel & Speath 1995) emphasise the importance of instilling the drops controlling the pressure.
- Instruct the patient about his drops and medication:
  - (a)  G. pilocarpine 1–2% 4 times a day;

## PATIENT INFORMATION LEAFLET No. 3

# GLAUCOMA DRAINAGE SURGERY

### Why do you need an operation?

Chronic glaucoma is a condition in which the pressure within the eye is higher than normal. The treatment that you are having now is not lowering the pressure sufficiently and the eye consultant feels that an operation to lower the pressure is now necessary.

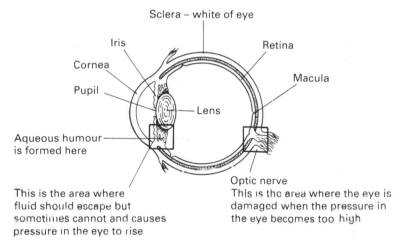

Sclera – white of eye
Iris
Retina
Cornea
Macula
Pupil
Lens
Aqueous humour is formed here
Optic nerve

This is the area where fluid should escape but sometimes cannot and causes pressure in the eye to rise

This is the area where the eye is damaged when the pressure in the eye becomes too high

### What does the operation involve?

Under anaesthetic a small cut is made in the outer layers of the eye and in the iris to allow the fluid inside the eye to drain out in a controlled fashion. This lowers the pressure in the eye. After a few weeks a small water blister forms and remains on the eye beneath the upper lid. This contains the draining fluid.

### When will you have your operation?

You will be advised of the waiting time for surgery and will be sent an appointment to attend a pre-admission clinic about two weeks before your operation. At this appointment you will see a nurse who will take all your personal details, a doctor will examine your eye, you will be given an explanation of the operation. You can also ask any questions that you may have during this appointment.

### What kind of anaesthetic will you have?

This depends on your preference and your general health. Your eye surgeon and anaesthetist will discuss the options with you. You may have a general

▶

**PATIENT INFORMATION LEAFLET No. 3** *continued*

anaesthetic, which involves being put to sleep throughout the operation. Alternatively you may have a local anaesthetic, which means that you are awake, but the eye and eyelids are numbed by an injection around the eye. The operation is therefore completely painfree. The injection will also blank out the vision during the operation, which takes about 30 minutes.

### How long will you be in hospital?

One or two nights in hospital is the usual length of stay and most people go home the day after their operation. However, occasionally you may need to stay longer.

### After your glaucoma operation

You can go back to your normal life, but remember the wound in your eye is delicate. Advice on various points is set out below.

### Drops

You should stop putting your glaucoma drops in the eye that has been operated upon, but these may need to be continued in the other eye if this is also affected by glaucoma. You will be given new drops to put in the operated eye for a few weeks. Detailed instructions for these drops will be given to you.

- Always wash your hands before and after instilling the drops to prevent infection.
- Always shake each bottle before instilling the drops.
- Don't let the bottle tip touch the eye.
- Keep using the drops until the doctor tells you to stop.
- Bring all of your eye drops to the outpatients clinic when you attend.

### Outpatients appointment

You will be seen in clinic one or two weeks after your operation, and then every four to six months thereafter.

### Pain or problems after your operation

If your eye aches, becomes sticky, or the vision deteriorates in the first two weeks following your discharge, telephone the ward for advice............ Thereafter, telephone Casualty for advice............

### Cleansing the eye

Cleanse the eye only if necessary. Close the eyelids and gently wipe the lids with a tissue damped with clean tap water.

### Work, housework, cooking and gardening

Avoid heavy lifting and straining for the first two weeks after the operation. Otherwise carry on as normal. Most people can return to work two weeks after the operation.

▶

---

**PATIENT INFORMATION LEAFLET No. 3 *continued***

**Driving**

It is best to avoid driving until after your first outpatients visit when you can ask the doctor if your vision is good enough to resume.

**At night**

For the first two weeks wear the protective eye shield which will be given to you.

**Bathing**

For the first two weeks avoid getting the eye wet or pressing on the eye. You may wash your hair, but avoid getting water and shampoo in the eye. If possible use a mild shampoo.

**Vision**

If your vision gradually deteriorates, first go to your own optician to see if your glasses need changing. If this is not the case ask your GP to refer you back to your eye consultant. If the deterioration is sudden please come to the Eye Casualty Department immediately.

Address:
Anytown Eye Unit
Anytown General Hospital
Any Road
Anytown
AN00 0AN

**Useful telephone numbers**

Ward . . . . . . . . . . . .
Casualty . . . . . . . . . . .
Outpatients . . . . . . . . . . .
Orthoptics . . . . . . . . . . .

---

    (b)   beta-blocker, e.g. levobunolol hydrochloride (Betagan) or timolol maleate (Timoptol) twice a day;

    (c)   acetazolamide tablets 250–500 mg 4 times a day or slow release twice a day.

## Laser treatment

- Prepare the patient for laser (see Section 3.2.20) trabeculoplasty which involves bombarding the trabecular meshwork with the laser. It is thought that scarring of the tissue stretches the meshwork and opens it up.

## Surgical treatment

- Admit patient to the ward.

- Prepare patient for operation, which is usually performed under a general anaesthetic.

  *Trabeculectomy* is the commonest type of drainage operation performed. This operation involves making a scleral flap and removing a strip of trabecular meshwork below this flap. The scleral flap is sutured back into place, but as this does not heal properly, it causes a fistula through which the aqueous can drain into the scleral vessels. The bulge over the scleral flap, lying under the conjunctiva, is called a 'bleb'.
- Give post-operative care.
  - (a)  Eye dressing.
    - (i)    A bleb should be noted under the conjunctiva.
    - (ii)   The anterior chamber will be shallow but should not be flat. If it is flat, the bleb is probably draining too much aqueous. A firm pad and bandage should be applied to seal the bleb.
  - (b)  Instillation of drops:
    - (i)    antibiotic;
    - (ii)   steroid;
    - (iii)  mydriatic.
- Discharge of patient. If he is receiving antagonistic drops to each eye he must be warned of the danger of a mix-up. The operated eye may be receiving a mydriatic and the unoperated eye a miotic as treatment for chronic glaucoma.

### Complications of trabeculectomy

*Early*

- Over-drainage.
- Under-drainage.
- Hyphaema.
- Aqueous misdirection into posterior segment of eye.

*Late*

- Subconjunctival fibrosis. Patients who have had long-term medical treatment prior to their surgery are more prone to fibrosis (Broadway 1994). Cytotoxic agents, such as 5-fluorouracil or mitomycin, given at the time of surgery or a few days post-operatively, can prevent this occurring (Skuta *et al.* 1992).
- Cataract formation due to surgical intervention.
- Infection as the bleb/fistula is only covered by conjunctiva.

### 10.7.3 Secondary glaucoma

Secondary glaucoma can be due to any of the following causes.

- *Conditions of the lens*
  - (a) Dislocation (see Section 11.5). The dislocated lens falls into the drainage angle or into the posterior chamber blocking the pupil.
  - (b) Cataract formation (see Section 11.2).
    - (i) The enlarged lens pushes forwards, blocking the pupil or angle This is called intumescence of the lens.
    - (ii) Lens material oozes out through the lens capsule clogging the angle. This is called phacolytic glaucoma.
- *Conditions of the uveal tract*
  - (a) Uveitis (see Section 9.5.2).
    - (i) Debris from the inflammation of the uveal tract may clog the drainage angle.
    - (ii) Pupil block caused by posterior synaechiae.
    - (iii) Permanent peripheral anterior synaechiae may develop from repeated attacks of uveitis.
  - (b) Tumours (see Section 9.5.3). Melanomas in the uveal tract cause raised intra-ocular pressure by volume replacement, encroachment on the angle or by blocking the vortex veins.
- *Trauma*
  - (a) Haemorrhage (hyphaema; see Section 14.9.1) into the anterior chamber. The blood in the anterior chamber clots in the angle.
  - (b) Angle recession.
  - (c) Corneal or limbal laceration (see Section 14.8.2). The anterior chamber is flattened and the angle closed by adherence of the anterior surface of the iris onto the posterior surface of the cornea.
- *Post-operative causes*
  - (a) Flat anterior chamber. Following intra-ocular surgery, aqueous may escape through the wound, causing a flat anterior chamber. If this persists, permanent anterior and posterior synaechiae may develop.
  - (b) Post-operative hyphaema. Blood clotting in the angle blocks the drainage channels.
- *Rubeosis iridis.* In diabetes mellitus and following occlusion of the central retinal vein, small blood vessels grow into the anterior surface of the iris (neovascularisation) and into the angle of the anterior chamber where they may block the drainage channels (thrombotic glaucoma). The new vessels may also cause a spontaneous hyphaema.
- *Steroids.* It is not clearly understood why long-term treatment with topical steroids cause a rise in intra-ocular pressure. Care must be taken in the use of topical steroids in patients with a family history of chronic glaucoma. Regular checks of intra-ocular pressure in these

patients and in long-term users of topical, and in some cases, systemic, steroids must be undertaken.

- *Thyroid eye disease.* Infiltration of the orbital fat and extra-ocular muscles pushes the globe forwards, causing pressure on the globe with a subsequent increase in intra-ocular pressure.

## Patient's needs

These are similar to those of primary acute glaucoma. A careful history must be taken because of the similarity in presenting signs and symptoms to primary acute glaucoma, and the other eye must be examined for depth of the anterior chamber.

## Nursing action

The cause of the secondary glaucoma, once diagnosed, is treated first. Therefore the nursing action will be that of the cause.

The intra-ocular pressure is reduced by medical treatment initially. Surgical intervention may be required if medical treatment fails to keep the intra-ocular pressure within normal limits. Nursing action will therefore be instruction of the patient on instillation of drops and taking medication, and administration of pre- and post-operative care when surgery is performed.

### 10.7.4   Buphthalmos/childhood glaucoma (ox-eye)

Buphthalmos is a rare congenital condition affecting 1 in 10 000 births and resulting in increased intra-ocular pressure caused by a defect or blockage of the drainage angle by an embryonic membrane. Occasionally the canal of Schlemm is absent. 40% have raised intra-ocular pressures *in utero*, 50% manifest in the first year of life and 10% manifest between the first and third year of life.

It is usually a bilateral condition, boys being more commonly affected than girls.

## Signs

- Large bulging eyes (Fig. 10.3). In childhood the sclera is more elastic than in the adult eye and the ever-increasing intra-ocular pressure stretches the sclera. It becomes thinned and appears blueish due to the pigment of the uveal tract showing through. The cornea also stretches. The enlargement of these two structures gives the child's eye the appearance of an ox-eye.
- Deep anterior chamber. The lens is pushed backwards by the increased pressure, thus forming a deep anterior chamber.

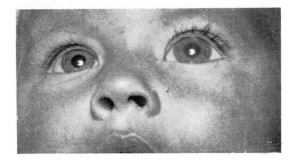

**Fig. 10.3** Buphthalmos.

- Large cornea. As the cornea is stretched, its diameter increases from a normal 9.0–11.5 cm to 12–14 cm. Tears may appear in Descemet's membrane.
- Deep cupping of the optic disc due to the raised intra-ocular pressure.
- The intra-ocular pressure will be between 25 mmHg and 45 mmHg.

## Patient's needs

- Relief of symptoms:
  - (a) lacrimation – child always appears to have running eyes and nose;
  - (b) photophobia – child often puts his arm over his eyes to shield them from the light;
  - (c) general irritability.
- Admission to hospital.
- General care of a child in hospital.

## Nursing action

- Admit the child to the ward.
- Give an explanation and reassurance to the parents. Involve them in as much of the child's care as possible.
- Prepare the patient for examination under anaesthetic. The following investigations are carried out:
  - (a) measurement of intra-ocular pressure;
  - (b) gonioscopy;
  - (c) ophthalmoscopy of optic disc;
  - (d) measurement of corneal diameter.

  These investigations are performed initially to diagnose the disease and thereafter at periodic intervals to assess success of treatment or progress of the disease.
- Give post-anaesthetic care following examination under anaesthesia.

- Administer pre-operative care if surgery is to be performed.
    (a) A goniotomy will be performed to open up the drainage channels by sweeping a goniotomy knife around the whole of the anterior chamber angle.
    (b) A drainage operation, such as a trabeculectomy, will be performed where the canal of Schlemm is absent or if the goniotomy fails to keep the intra-ocular pressure within normal limits. A combined procedure of trabeculotomy and trabeculectomy may be more successful than trabeculectomy alone (Elder 1994).
- Give post-operative care:
    (a) instillation of antibiotic and/or steroid drops – a mydriatic may be used;
    (b) observation of the 'bleb' and depth of anterior chamber following trabeculectomy (see Section 10.7.2).
    If the glaucoma is unilateral, amblyopia must be prevented in that eye (see Section 13.3). Patching of the unaffected eye will be instituted to encourage the child to use the glaucomatous eye.

### Prognosis

The prognosis depends on when the disease became manifest (see above). The earlier the disease is present, the worse the prognosis and visual impairment may be severe.

### Complications

- Corneal/scleral perforation due to the thinning of those structures. Perforation may occur with the least trauma.
- Exposure keratitis due to the lids being unable to lubricate the enlarged cornea adequately.

A bandage contact lens can be used to prevent and treat both these conditions.

### 10.7.5   Juvenile glaucoma

Juvenile glaucoma is associated with neurofibromatosis, Sturge–Weber syndrome, rubella and aniridia. It presents later than buphthalmos and behaves like chronic open-angle glaucoma. Hence care of the patient is similar.

# 11  The Lens

## 11.1  INTRODUCTION

### 11.1.1  Structure of the lens

The lens is a biconvex, transparent, avascular structure with no nerve supply (Fig. 11.1). It measures 9 mm by 4 mm in diameter. The lens lies behind the iris and in front of the vitreous. It is supported by the zonules or suspensory ligaments which attach it to the ciliary processes.

The lens has an elastic capsule which enables it to change shape during accommodation (see Section 9.3). This capsule is semipermeable to water and electrolytes. The lens receives its nourishment from the aqueous.

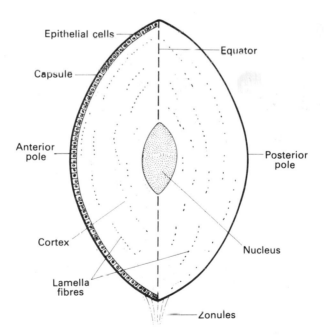

**Fig. 11.1** Cross-section of lens structure. (Reproduced with permission from *Ophthalmic Nursing*, Smith & Nachazel (1980), published by Little, Brown and Company.)

The anterior surface has a single layer of epithelial cells. The anterior pole is less convex than the posterior pole.

The *cortex* of the lens is composed of a gelatinous substance and lamella fibres which are arranged in layers like an onion and originate from the anterior epithelial layer. These fibres are continually being produced so that the lens enlarges slowly throughout life. Where the lamella fibres meet end-to-end, suture lines are formed. In the nucleus these are Y-shaped and when viewed with the slit lamp, can be seen to be erect anteriorly, i.e. Y, and inverted posteriorly, i.e ʎ.

The *nucleus* is composed of sclerosed lens fibres. These are old cortical fibres that cannot be cast off and are therefore massed together in the centre as the nucleus. The nucleus grows in size and is harder than the cortex.

### 11.1.2   Composition of the lens

65% water
35% protein
In addition, there are trace minerals, the most important being sodium, potassium and calcium.

### 11.1.3   Function of the lens

The function of the lens is to focus light rays on the retina by 'accommodation' (see Section 9.3). After the age of 45 years, the lens has become so solid that it gradually loses its ability to change shape. This means that the lens cannot accommodate for near vision, a condition called presbyopia. Spectacles are therefore needed for reading. The presbyopia slowly increases until the age of 70 years, those affected requiring increasingly stronger lenses in reading glasses.

## 11.2   CATARACT

A cataract is an opacity of the lens. The lens is a delicate structure and any insult on it causes absorption of water, resulting in the lens becoming opaque.

Cataracts can be defined according to their type, location and degree.

### 11.2.1   The types of cataract

- Congenital.
- Familial.
- Senile.
- Traumatic.

- Toxic.
- Secondary to existing eye disease.
- Associated with systemic disease.

### 11.2.2 Location of the opacity

Cataracts can occur in different parts of the lens:

- anterior pole cataract;
- posterior pole cataract;
- nuclear cataract;
- cortical cataract;
- lamellar cataract.

### 11.2.3 Degrees of cataract

- Immature cataract – part of the lens is opaque.
- Mature cataract – the whole lens is opaque and may be swollen (intumescent) (Fig. 11.2).
- Hypermature cataract – the lens becomes dehydrated because water has escaped from the lens, leaving an opaque lens and wrinkled capsule.
- Phakolytic lens – lens matter leaks out causing uveitis and secondary glaucoma. Cataracts should be extracted before this situation arises.

The mature and hypermature cataract can be viewed through the pupil. An immature cataract can be seen when viewed with a slit lamp.

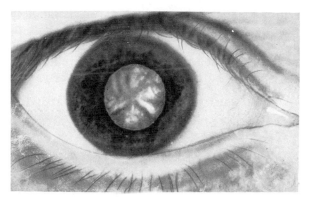

**Fig. 11.2** Mature cataract.

### 11.2.4   Congenital cataract

**Causes**

- Rubella or malnutrition in the first trimester of pregnancy results in a lamellar cataract in the baby.
- Abnormal development of the eye in the fetus causes pressure on the anterior pole, resulting in an anterior pole cataract.
- A tag of hyaloid membrane remaining from fetal life can result in a posterior pole cataract. (The hyaloid membrane runs from the retina to the lens during fetal life.)
- Metabolic disturbance such as galactosaemia results in a nuclear cataract.

**Signs of a cataract in a baby or child**

- A white pupil may be noted by the parents or health visitor. It may be unilateral or bilateral. The cause of the white pupil must be diagnosed to differentiate it from the more serious condition retinoblastoma (see Section 12.6.7).
- The parents may notice that the child does not see well.
- A squint will indicate that there is a lesion in the visual pathway preventing the sight from developing. The cause again must be differentiated from a retinoblastoma.

It is important that cataracts are removed as soon as possible to prevent amblyopia occurring (see Section 13.3). This is especially important if the cataracts are bilateral and dense, when extraction should be carried out before the baby is two months old.

The rule of thumb is that if the fundus can be seen, then light must be reaching the retina. Amblyopia (see Section 13.3) will therefore not develop. Removal of the lens will itself cause amblyopia as the light rays are not directed onto the retina by the lens. Compliance with aphakic correction (see Sections 11.3.1 and 11.3.2) is therefore very important in these children.

### 11.2.5   Familial cataract

Familial cataracts can occur, but they are rare, affecting the 30–40 year age group.

### 11.2.6   Senile cataract

Senile cataracts occur in patients over the age of 60 years. They result from sclerosis of the lens due to a degenerative process. The rate of progression varies. It is usually a bilateral condition, one eye being affected before the other.

The cataract is either nuclear or cortical.

- A *nuclear cataract* affects the central lens and takes on a brown colour. In this instance the patient sees better in dim light when the pupil is dilated and the light rays can enter the eye around the central opacity. Mydriatics can be given to dilate the pupil and give some vision around the cataract.
- A *cortical cataract* affects the periphery of the lens and looks white. This type of cataract can produce a uni-ocular diplopia as the opacity splits the light rays. Vision is usually better in bright light when the pupil constricts and so reduces the peripheral distortion.

### 11.2.7 Traumatic cataract – see Section 14.10.1

### 11.2.8 Toxic cataract

Toxic substances can affect the metabolism of the lens and cause opacity formation. Radiation and drugs such as topical steroids have this effect.

### 11.2.9 Cataracts secondary to existing eye diseases

Glaucoma, retinitis pigmentosa, retinal detachments, retinopathies, choroiditis and uveitis upset the metabolism of the lens, causing cataract formation. The opacities form in the posterior subcapsular area, eventually involving the entire lens.

### 11.2.10 Cataracts associated with systemic disease

Some systemic diseases cause an upset in the metabolism of the lens, causing, in the main, posterior subcapsular opacities.

- *Diabetes mellitus.* The increased glucose level in the aqueous is taken up by the lens disturbing its metabolism. Cataracts can occur with rapid onset in juvenile diabetics, the lens becoming completely opaque within several weeks. In older diabetics the opacities are nuclear, posterior subcapsular or cortical in nature and take longer to develop.
- *Hypoparathyroidism.* Cataract formation from this cause is usually seen after the removal of the parathyroid glands during thyroid gland removal. It can be idiopathic. Low calcium levels disturb the lens metabolism.
- *Atopic disease.* Dermatological conditions such as eczema and scleroderma can, when severe and widespread, cause cataract formation.

## 11.2.11  Visual effects of a cataract

Patients with cataracts complain of gradually fading vision and a variety of visual disturbances. Depending on the site of the cataract, as has been mentioned above, they may be able to see better in dim or bright conditions. Some complain of dazzling bright lights due to irregular refraction of rays through the opacities in the lens. Some patients experience uniocular diplopia. Posterior capsular opacities cause difficulty in near vision, leaving distance vision unaffected.

**Patient's needs** (see Patient Information Leaflet No. 4)

Cataract extraction is commonly performed as a day case.

* Pre-assessment.
* Keratometry and A-scan (see Section 3.2.26) for estimating strength of intra-ocular lens.
* Pre- and post-operative care.

**Nursing action**

* Prepare the patient for a general or local anaesthetic which may be topical and periocular or topical and subconjunctival (Anderson 1995). The pupil will be dilated before surgery.
* Give post-operative care. *Eye care*:
    (a)  on examination the conjunctiva will be mildly injected:
        (i)   the cornea should be clear;
        (ii)  the anterior chamber should be deep and quiet;
        (iii) the pupil should be central – it may still be dilated from the effects of the pre-operative mydriatics and slightly eccentric initially;
    (b)  if a posterior chamber intra-ocular lens is *in situ*, its reflection may be noted through the pupil;
    (c)  an antibiotic and steroid drop will be instilled;
    (d)  cataract surgery is usually considered fairly pain free. However, Allen & Oberle (1993) found that 15% of the patients in their study experienced severe pain on the first post-operative day;
    (e)  post-operative information (see Patient Information Leaflet No. 4) should be given. Allen *et al.* (1992) discovered in their research that no patient received complete information. Phacoemulsification requires less stringent post-operative restrictions, swimming and driving being the two main activities to be avoided until advised otherwise, usually at the first post-operative outpatient visit.

If glasses need to be prescribed, this will be carried out 2–6 weeks after surgery.

## PATIENT INFORMATION LEAFLET No. 4

# CATARACTS

### What is a cataract?

A cataract is a misting or opacity of the lens of the eye. It prevents light entering properly and causes dimness of vision. It can also cause dazzle in bright light. Most cataracts are caused by the body's normal ageing process but occasionally they are caused by injury, diabetes or drugs. They can occur, although rarely, in babies due to faulty development of the lens.

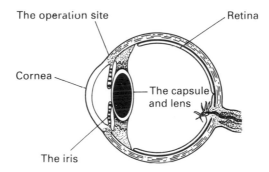

### How can a cataract be treated?

Mild cataracts may not require treatment, or a simple change in spectacles may improve the vision. Your optician can advise you on this point. If your vision is becoming so impaired that it is causing difficulties in your daily living (including driving), then it might be time for an operation to remove the cataract in order to restore your vision. Your eye surgeon will advise you about this. The operation is short and simple and in most cases the lens containing the cataract is replaced by a plastic lens implanted inside the eye. This lens is painless and remains in the eye for the rest of your life.

### When will you have your operation?

You will be advised about the waiting time for your surgery and will be sent an appointment to attend a pre-admission clinic about two weeks before your operation. At this clinic you will see a nurse who will take all your personal details, a doctor who will examine your eye, and you will be given an explanation of the operation. You can also ask any questions that you may have during this appointment.

### What kind of anaesthetic will you have?

This depends on your preference and your general health. Your eye surgeon

▶

**PATIENT INFORMATION LEAFLET No. 4** *continued*

and the anaesthetist will discuss the options with you. You may have a general anaesthetic which involves being put to sleep throughout the operation. Alternatively, you may have a local anaesthetic which means that you are awake, but the eye and eyelids are numbed by an injection around the eye. The operation is therefore completely pain free. The injection will also blank out the vision during the operation, which takes about 30 minutes.

**How long will you be in hospital?**

One or two nights in hospital is the usual length of stay and most people go home the day after their operation. Occasionally you will need to stay longer. Some people may have their operation carried out as a day case and no overnight stay is necessary. If you are interested in having your operation as a day case patient a separate information leaflet is available.

**After your cataract**

You can go back to your normal life immediately but remember that the wound in your eye is delicate. Advice on various points is set out below.

**Drops**

You will be given drops to put in your eye for a few weeks after the operation. Detailed instructions will be given to you.

- Always wash your hands before and after instilling the drops to prevent infection.
- Always shake each bottle before instilling the drops.
- Don't let the bottle tip touch the eye.
- Keep on using the drops until the eye doctor tells you to stop.
- Please bring all drops to the clinic when you attend.

**Outpatients appointments**

You will normally be seen two or three times after your operation, usually one or two weeks after surgery and again about six weeks later. If all is well you will then be discharged.

**Pain or problems after your operation**

If your eye aches, becomes sticky, or the vision deteriorates in the first two weeks following your discharge, telephone the ward for advice . . . . . . . . . . . . Thereafter, telephone Casualty for advice . . . . . . . . . . . .

**Cleansing the eye**

Cleanse the eye only if necessary. Close the eyelids and gently wipe the lids with a tissue dampened with clean tap-water.

**Work, housework, cooking and gardening**

Avoid heavy lifting and straining for the first two weeks. Otherwise carry on as normal taking care not to knock the eye. Most people can return to work two weeks after the operation.

▶

## PATIENT INFORMATION LEAFLET No. 4 *continued*

### Driving

It is best to avoid driving, until after your first outpatient visit when you can ask the doctor if your vision is good enough to resume.

### At night

For the first week wear the protective eye shield which will be given to you.

### Bathing

You may wash your hair but avoid getting shampoo or water in the eye. If possible, use a mild shampoo.

### Glasses

After your operation your vision may initially be blurred. You can wear your present spectacles (or dark glasses) if they help, but you will probably need a change of spectacles about two months after your operation. You will need to go to your optician for these.

### Stitches

The stitches remain in your eye. Occasionally they may break and cause a scratchy feeling in your eye. Please come to the Eye Casualty Department if this occurs. Sometimes it is necessary to remove some or all of the stitches after your wound has healed, 6–8 weeks after your operation. This is done in the Eye Unit Outpatient Department and is painless.

### Vision

If your vision gradually deteriorates, first go to your own optician to see if your glasses need changing. If this is not the case ask your GP to refer you back to your eye consultant. If the deterioration is sudden please come to the Eye Casualty Department immediately.

Address:
Anytown Eye Unit
Anytown General Hospital
Any Road
Anytown
AN00 0AN

### Useful telephone numbers

Ward . . . . . . . . . . . .
Casualty . . . . . . . . . . . .
Outpatients . . . . . . . . . . . .
Orthoptics . . . . . . . . . . . .

## 11.2.12   Cataract operations

The approach is via a limbal incision under a conjunctival flap or via a peripheral corneal incision.

### Needling or lens aspiration

Needling or lens aspiration is performed on an infant or child under the age of 15 years. The cortex and nucleus of the lens are irrigated out through an incision in the anterior lens capsule, leaving the posterior capsule behind in order to prevent vitreous prolapse. At this age, the lens matter is soft enough to be aspirated.

The posterior lens capsule left behind often scleroses causing visual impairment when a *capsulotomy* will be performed using the Yag laser.

### 'Lensectomy' (Phacofragmentation)

Lensectomy involves removing the entire lens and capsule and an anterior segment of the vitreous using specialised equipment. It is used for congenital cataracts and has the advantage of not requiring future capsulotomies.

### Intracapsular lens extraction

In an intracapsular lens extraction, the entire lens plus its capsule is removed. An enzyme chymotripsin is introduced into the eye to dissolve the zonular fibres. The lens is then free of its attachments and can be removed from the eye by forceps or the cryoprobe. An anterior chamber intra-ocular lens will be implanted (see below). This procedure is rarely employed nowadays, but the nurse may encounter patients having had this type of surgery in the past.

### Extracapsular lens extraction

In an extracapsular lens extraction the anterior lens capsule, the cortex and nucleus are removed, leaving the posterior lens capsule in place. The type of incision made in the anterior lens capsule may vary, e.g. endo-capsular, capsulorhexis. Following this type of surgery, cortical matter may proliferate on the intact posterior capsule, a condition requiring capsulotomy (see above). A posterior chamber intra-ocular lens will be implanted.

### Phacoemulsification

With phacoemulsification the lens is broken down by ultrasonic vibrations. This technique is becoming increasingly popular as it reduces the risk of expulsive haemorrhage and post-operative astigmatism (McNicholl 1995) as the incision is smaller (3 mm) than that used in the operations described above. Suturing the wound is not required if it is properly sealed. A foldable intra-ocular lens is positioned in the posterior chamber. Alternatively, the wound is enlarged to accommodate a non-foldable lens implant.

## 11.3 APHAKIA

### 11.3.1 Correction of aphakia

Aphakia is the absence of the lens. Without the lens the eye becomes very hypermetropic, requiring some kind of lens replacement to enable the patient to see adequately. The only people who do not require correction of the aphakia are those who are very miopic in whom the absence of the lens causes the light rays to focus on the retina.

Aphakia causes loss of accommodation so patients will need correction for both near and distance vision. Following surgery, a degree of astigmatism will result, requiring correction as well.

### 11.3.2 Types of correction

Aphakia can be corrected using glasses, contact lenses or intra-ocular lenses

### Aphakic glasses

These glasses are rarely used nowadays. They may be used in babies when contact lenses are unsuitable.

### Contact lenses

Contact lenses are increasingly being superceded by intra-ocular lenses (see below) but nurses may meet patients who have had earlier surgery and wear contact lenses to correct their aphakia.

#### Use (in aphakia)

- Unilateral or bilateral aphakia.

#### Advantages

- They can be used for unilateral aphakia.

- They give a full field of vision.
- They can be used in babies and children.
- They only cause 7% magnification.

*Disadvantages* (also see Appendix 2)

- Patients have to become accustomed to wearing contact lenses; some may find them intolerable.
- Corneal abrasions and infections can result from contact lens wearing and from unclean lenses.
- Patients with arthritis cannot manipulate them, but extended-wear lenses overcome this problem.
- The lenses are easily lost.
- They need scrupulous cleaning, especially soft contact lenses.
- Bilateral aphakics may find difficulty in putting the first lens in because of poor sight in the other eye. Again, extended-wear lenses can overcome this.
- They are expensive for those who are not eligible to have them supplied by the NHS.
- They may not be suitable to be worn in some occupations, e.g. when working in a dusty environment.

**Intra-ocular lenses** (Fig. 11.3)

*Uses*

- Unilateral and bilateral aphakia.

*Types*

There are many named lenses made by different companies. Those listed below are just some examples.

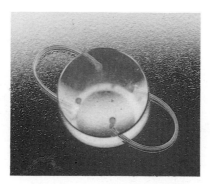

**Fig. 11.3** An intra-ocular lens (IOL).

- *Anterior chamber lenses*, e.g. Choyce, Severin. These lenses are placed in the anterior chamber of the eye following an intra-capsular extraction or if the posterior capsule ruptures during surgery.
- *Posterior chamber lenses*, e.g. Sinsky. These lenses are inserted into the posterior chamber of the eye following an extracapsular extraction, fitting into the posterior lens capsule which has been left behind. Newer lenses are being manufactured with 'laser ridges' to keep the lens away from the capsule to prevent the lens being damaged by the laser beam during a capsulotomy.
- *Folding lenses*, e.g. Allergan. These lenses can be used with phacoemulsification and are placed in the posterior capsule.

## Advantages

- Full field of vision is attained 24 hours a day.
- They can be inserted at any time after the initial cataract extraction.
- No manual dexterity or manipulation is required on behalf of the wearer.
- They are suitable for workers in industry or those in a humid environment/occupation.
- Vision is good even without glasses. Bifocal intra-ocular lenses are available (Pearce 1996), but as yet are not used very often.
- Posterior chamber intra-ocular lenses have been successfully implanted in children (Brady *et al.* 1995).
- Heparin coated lenses can be used in patients who have repeated attacks of uveitis.

## Disadvantages

- They can cause uveitis and glaucoma.
- They can dislocate.
- Anterior chamber lenses may cause bullous keratopathy.

## Pre-operative investigations

- Biometry (see Section 3.2.27).
- Keratometry (see Section 3.2.26).
- *The 'B' Scan.* The 'B' Scan is an ultrasound scan used before cataract extractions. It gives a three-dimensional picture of the eye, showing up any abnormality in the media, such as a retinal detachment or tumour. This examination is necessary because the ophthalmologist is unable to examine the fundus through an opaque lens. If a tumour or retinal detachment were noted, the lens extraction might not take place, as no improvement in vision would occur.
- *Laser interferometre* projects a Snellen chart on to the retina to determine

the visual potential in an eye with dense lens opacities (Vaughan 1995). If the visual potential is not tested for, a patient may not have good post-operative visual acuity due to undiagnosed age-related macular degeneration (see Section 12.7).


## 11.4   COMPLICATIONS OF CATARACT EXTRACTION

Modern cataract surgery gives good visual results and is a relatively safe procedure (Powe *et al.* 1994). However, complications do occur (Powe *et al.* 1994):

*Early* (in order of occurrence)

• Zonular/posterior capsule rupture.
• Lens dislocation into vitreous.
• Vitreous loss.
• Wound gape/iris prolapse.
• Hyphaema.
• Vitreous/choroidal haemorrhage.
• Hypopyon.
• Endophthalmitis.


*Late* (in order of occurrence)

• Posterior capsular opacification.
• Uveitis.
• Cystoid macular oedaema.
• Raised intra-ocular pressure.
• Dislocated/malpositioned intra-ocular lens.
• Retinal detachment.
• Bullous keratopathy.


## 11.5   DISLOCATED LENS

A total dislocation of the lens or a partial dislocation (subluxation) can occur.

This can be a result of trauma, it may be hereditary, or be associated with certain syndromes such as Marfan's syndrome. Vision will be blurred, but the degree of visual disturbance depends on the degree of dislocation. A partially dislocated lens can usually be seen through the pupil. A cataract may develop in the lens.

A dislocated lens can cause uveitis or glaucoma by blocking either the posterior or anterior chambers.

If no complications occur, dislocated lenses are best left untreated. If complications do occur, treatment should be given to the complications before cataract extraction is attempted, as surgery in these instances is difficult.

# 12 The Retina, Optic Nerve and Vitreous

## 12.1 THE RETINA

The retina is composed of ten layers: one epithelial layer and nine neural layers. There is a potential space between the epithelial layer and neural layers which is significant in retinal detachment. The retina extends from the ora serrata anteriorly to the optic disc posteriorly where the nerve fibres leave the eye as the optic nerve.

### 12.1.1 Ten layers of the retina (Fig. 12.1)

(1) The *epithelial layer* lies at the posterior of the structure beneath the choroid and contains varying amounts of melanin pigment. It absorbs light which is not picked up by the rods and cones.
(2) The *receptor layer* contains the rods and cones, which are the two main types of nerve endings in the retina.
   The *rods*, numbering about 120 million, are situated mainly at the periphery of the retina. They function in dim light.
   The *cones*, numbering around 7 million, are situated at the centre of the retina and are concentrated, in particular, in the fovea of the macula. They function in bright light, pick up colours and make detailed vision possible.
(3) The *external limiting membrane* is like a sheet of wire netting and has a supportive function.
(4) The *outer nuclear layer* contains the nuclei of the rods and cones.
(5) The *outer plexiform layer* contains the axons of the rods and cones and the dendrites of the bipolar cells.
(6) The *inner nuclear layer* contains the nuclei of the bipolar cells.
(7) The *inner plexiform layer* contains the axons of bipolar cells and the dendrites of the ganglion cells.
(8) The *ganglion cell layer* contains the nuclei of the ganglion cells.
(9) The *nerve fibre layer* contains the axons of the ganglion cells which

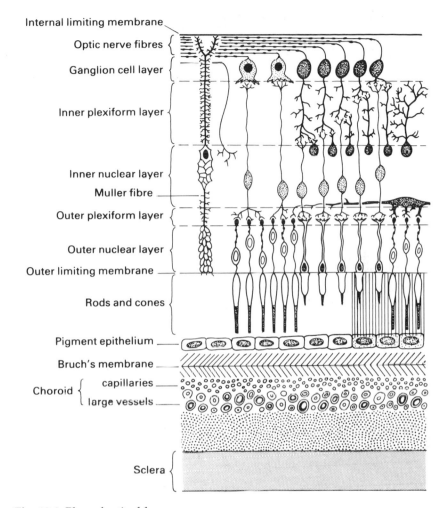

Internal limiting membrane

Optic nerve fibres

Ganglion cell layer

Inner plexiform layer

Inner nuclear layer

Muller fibre

Outer plexiform layer

Outer nuclear layer

Outer limiting membrane

Rods and cones

Pigment epithelium

Bruch's membrane

Choroid { capillaries

large vessels

Sclera

**Fig. 12.1** Plan of retinal layers.

pass through the optic disc and lamina cibrosa to become continuous with the optic nerve.

(10)   The *internal limiting membrane* has a supportive function.

Layers 2–10 are known as the 'neural layers'.

### 12.1.2   Areas of the retina

- *Ora serrata* – the anterior termination of the retina where the retinal pigment epithelial layer continues forwards to become the ciliary epithelium. The neural layer of the retina ends at the ora serrata.
- *Macula* (Fig. 12.2) – an area of the retina 1.5 mm in diameter situated

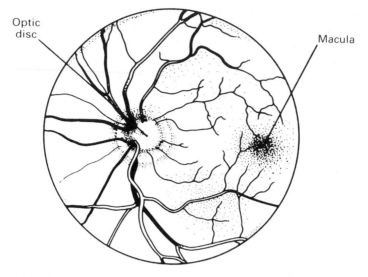

Optic
disc

Macula

**Fig. 12.2** Ophthalmoscopic view of the normal retina. (Reproduced with permission from Vaughan, D.G. & Asbury, T. (1983) *General Ophthalmology* (10th edn), Appleton & Lange.)

3 mm to the temporal side of the optic disc. It contains a high concentration of cones. In its centre is the *fovea centralis*, a slight depression where only cones are present. The other layers of the retina are absent here, causing a depression and making it thinner than the rest of the retina. The macula is the region of the retina where central precise vision takes place. It is not completely developed until 6 months after birth. No blood vessels cross the macula and it receives its blood supply entirely from the choriocapillaries.

- *Optic disc* (Fig. 12.2) – the area of the retina where the axons of the ganglion cells leave the eye through the lamina cribrosa to become continuous with the optic nerve. It therefore contains no nerve cells, so that vision cannot take place here. This is known as the 'blind spot'. The central retinal artery and vein pass through the optic disc. Its blood supply is from the posterior ciliary artery, a branch of the temporal artery.

### 12.1.3  Blood supply

The outer layers of the retina are supplied by the choriocapillaries of the choroid. The inner layers of the retina are supplied by the central retinal artery. The central retinal vein drains the venous blood.

### 12.1.4  Function of the retina

The retinal nerve cells pick up and transmit impulses from light rays reaching the retina. These impulses then travel via the optic pathways to the visual cortex where they are interpreted as sight (see Fig. 12.3). As light rays travel in straight lines they will fall on the diagonally opposite area of the retina from the object in view; for example, the light rays from an object viewed superiorly will fall on the inferior area of the retina. The same happens on the horizontal plane. The brain converts the image so it appears the right way up.

## 12.2 THE OPTIC NERVE

The optic nerve runs from the optic disc through the optic foramen to the optic chiasma where it becomes the optic tract. It is 5 cm in length. It is surrounded by pia, arachnoid and dura. Its blood supply is via the ophthalmic artery and vein.

### 12.2.1 The optic pathways (Fig. 12.3)

The optic nerve leaves each eye, passing through the optic foramen to the optic chiasma. From there the fibres from the left-hand side of each eye

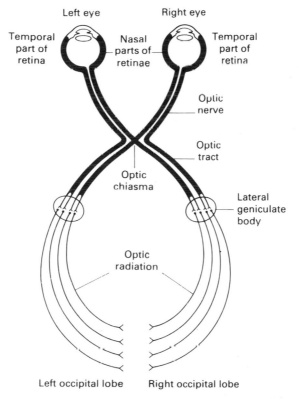

**Fig. 12.3** Visual pathways. (Reprinted from Darling & Thorpe *Ophthalmic Nursing* (1981) Fig. 21, p. 74 by permission of the publisher Baillière Tindall Limited, London.)

travel in the left-hand side of the brain and the right-hand fibres travel in the right-hand side of the brain. Thus the nasal fibres in the left eye cross at the chiasma to travel on the right side and the nasal fibres of the right eye cross to travel on the left side. The temporal fibres of each eye stay on their respective side. From the optic chiasma the fibres travel in the optic tracts to the lateral geniculate bodies where they pass into the optic radiations. From there the fibres pass to the visual area of the occipital cortex where sight is interpreted.

## 12.3   THE VITREOUS

The vitreous fills the vitreous chamber which is the posterior segment of the eye lying between the lens and the retina. (Not to be confused with the posterior chamber.)

It is a semi-gelatinous, transparent substance having no blood or nerve supply.

### 12.3.1   Composition

98%–99%    water
 1%–2%     hyaluronic acid
           collagen fibres

### 12.3.2   Attachments

The vitreous is attached more firmly to the underlying retina at the ora serrata and around the optic disc. Elsewhere it lies loosely against the retina. Sometimes it attaches itself to blood vessels, which could bleed if the vitreous pulled on them.

### 12.3.3   Functions of the vitreous

- Refractions of light. The light rays travel in a converged manner through the vitreous towards the retina.
- It maintains the shape of the eye. If it were lost, the eye would collapse. Vitreous cannot be replaced naturally by the eye.

## 12.4   COLOUR VISION

The cones in the retina can be divided into three types: red, blue and green. Each of these types is sensitive to different light rays. The red absorb long waves, the green mid-length waves and the blue short waves. These differing wave lengths or a combination of them are interpreted as colour.

## 12.5  RHODOPSIN

Rhodopsin is a photosensitive chemical present in the rods in the retina. In low-intensity light rhodopsin breaks down, taking a few moments to work and enabling the eye to adapt to dim light. When changing from low intensity light to bright light, it takes a few seconds to bleach the rhodopsin and enable the eye to adapt to bright light. Vitamin A is necessary for rhodopsin to function, thus a deficiency of vitamin A can lead to night blindness.

## 12.6  CONDITIONS OF THE RETINA

### 12.6.1  Retinal detachment

Retinal detachment is a misnomer because it is not a detachment of the retina from the underlying choroid. It is, in fact, a separation of the epithelial layer from the neural layers of the retina. Because of the potential space between the first layer and the rest of the retina, it can become separated as a result of disease or trauma.

**Causes**

The neural retina can be either pulled, pushed or floated off the underlying epithelial layer.

- *Pulled off.* The neural retina is pulled off the epithelial layer by vitreous traction. Vitreous traction occurs when new blood vessels have grown into the vitreous. The fragile vessels bleed and fibrous tissue forms in the healing process. These fibrous bands contract, pulling the neural layer away. Conditions causing this type of detachment are diabetes mellitus, retinopathy of prematurity, retinal haemorrhage and vitreous haemorrhage.

- *Pushed off.* A lesion behind the retina pushes the retina forwards, causing fluid or exudate to separate the layers of the retina. Conditions causing this type of detachment are choroidal tumours, choroidal haemorrhage, choroiditis and retinopathies.

- *Floated off.* If a tear or hole appears in the retina, subretinal fluid or vitreous fluid enters the hole, floating the neural layers off the epithelial layer. Tears in the retina occur following trauma, in high myopes, retinal degeneration (see Section 12.6.6) and aphakia. The tears usually occur in the periphery or equator of the retina.

**Patient's needs**

- Relief of symptoms:
  (a)  flashing lights (photopsia) – caused by the separating layers of the retina stimulating the rods and cones;
  (b)  floaters – a sudden increase in the number of floaters in the vision, or a shower of floaters, occurs. These are small haemorrhages, usually from retinal vessels;
  (c)  field loss – as the retina separates, the affected part causes loss of vision in the corresponding visual field. It must be remembered that the visual field loss is opposite to the detachment; for example, if the upper half of the retina is detached, the visual loss would be the lower half of the visual field. It is important to prevent the macula from detaching, as the visual prognosis following this occurrence is not good. The separated macula will be denied its blood supply from the choriocapillaries and will therefore become anoxic. Unfortunately the commonest site for a detachment is in the superior temporal area causing an inferior nasal visual field loss. This area of the visual field is occluded to some extent by the nose, the vision in the other eye compensating for it. Therefore field loss in this area is not noticed as quickly as field loss in another area. Also a superior detachment can progress more rapidly due to gravity and the danger of a macular detachment is therefore greater.
- Admission to hospital for bed rest and pre- and post-operative care.
- Surgery to re-attach the retina.

**Nursing action**

- Inform the doctor of the patient's history and type of visual loss.
- Instil prescribed mydriatic drops for ophthalmoscopic examination of the fundus.
- Admit patient to the ward.
- Give pre-operative care.
  (a)  Bed rest, to prevent further detachment occurring.
  (b)  Dependent positioning. This is decided, to some extent, by the doctor's wishes and the site of the detachment. The rationale is to position the patient so that the detachment lies dependently against its underlying epithelial layer, encouraging the subretinal fluid to be absorbed and re-attachment to occur.
  (c)  Instil prescribed mydriatic drops regularly to maintain mydriasis so that a good fundal examination can be carried out. This is performed using an indirect ophthalmoscope and a 20 dioptre lens to obtain an accurate diagram of the retina, including tears, holes, detached and attached areas, and the presence of sub-

retinal fluid. This helps the surgeon at the time of operation. The other eye is also dilated and inspected. Retinopathies, degenerations, and myopia can affect both eyes. Problems in the other eye must be noted and treated if present, often using laser or cryotherapy prophylactically.

- Give post-operative care.
  - (a) Eye care:
    - (i) the lids and conjunctiva are usually swollen following retinal detachment because of the amount of movement of the eye that is necessary during surgery;
    - (ii) the cornea must be noted for its clarity; if it is cloudy, this could indicate ischaemia of the anterior segment of the eye caused by the encirclement band being too tight (see below);
    - (iii) the pupil will remain dilated;
    - (iv) antibiotic, mydriatic and steroid drops, non-steroidal anti-inflammatory drops may be prescribed.
  - (b) General care. The patient may be nursed in a dependent position following surgery. This is especially important following vitrectomy, when the injected gas or air bubble must be uppermost to put pressure on the detached retina (see below). Analgesia will need to be given regularly as ocular pain will be experienced by most patients. It must be ascertained that the cause of pain is not raised pressure due to anterior segment ischaemia (see above).

### Types of retinal detachment surgery

The eye is not opened for detachment surgery, the approach being from the outside over the sclera, apart from a vitrectomy in which case the eye is opened.

- *Cryotherapy, laser* or *photocoagulation* is performed to seal holes or tears by setting up a local inflammatory reaction and thereby preventing fluid seeping between the retinal layers. Holes and tears, if present, must be sealed during detachment operations for this surgery to be successful.
- *Plombage* or *scleral buckling*. A silastic sponge or 'plomb' – a small square of inert material – is sutured onto the sclera over the site of the hole, causing an indentation and bringing the separated layers of the retina together.
- *Encirclement*. A silicone band is positioned around the globe, underneath the extra-ocular muscles. This enables greater indentation to occur and is used where there is a large area of detachment or multiple holes.
- *Drainage of subretinal fluid* must be performed at the time of each of

the above surgical procedures to allow the separated layers to realign.
- *Vitrectomy* may be performed in certain circumstances (see below).

## Complications

### *Early*

- Subretinal fluid may continue to accumulate between the layers of the retina. This must be removed if spontaneous reabsorption does not occur in order to prevent further detachment occurring and to aid re-attachment.
- Ischaemia of the anterior segment of the eye following encirclement if the band is too tight.

### *Late*

- Infection of the plomb or band, in which case removal is necessary.
- Extrusion of the plomb. The plomb may become loose and work its way to the surface under the conjunctiva.

## Vitrectomy

Vitrectomy is performed for the following conditions:

- giant tears;
- retinal detachment with scar formation;
- fibrovascular tissue in diabetic retinopathy;
- dislocated lens;
- foreign body in posterior segment;
- penetrating injury;
- vitreous tap for microscopy.

Vitreous cannot be replaced naturally. One of the following substances is used as replacement material:

(1) *Gas*, e.g. $SF_6$ (sulphur hexafluoride), $C_3F_8$ (perfluoropropane). The patient cannot see through the gas until it has been absorbed and this takes 2 to 3 weeks.
(2) *Silicone oil*. The patient can see through the oil but it makes the eye hypermetropic. Silicone oil is not absorbed.
(3) *Air*. This is absorbed within 24 to 36 hours.
(4) *Gas and air mixture.*
(5) $C_{10}F_{18}$ (perfluorodecaline). This is a heavy liquid which is not absorbed.

Aqueous will gradually fill the vitreous chamber to replace the above substances as they are absorbed (except the oil and $C_{10}F_{18}$).

In order to carry out a vitrectomy, the vitreous chamber/posterior segment is approached via three entry ports at the ora serrata (pars plana) to prevent damage to the retina. The vitreous is broken up and aspirated out of the eye. All instruments entering the vitreous chamber are 27 gauge in size. Up to 90% of the vitreous can be removed.

**Complications of vitrectomy surgery**

- Cataract formation.
- Oil in the anterior segment.
- Emulsified oil in the anterior chamber or between the main bubble and the retina.
- The bubble will expand when flying. Patients are advised not to fly if the bubble is more than 10% of the volume of the eye.

**Post-operative nursing care** (in addition to that mentioned above)

(a) Eye care. Observe the entry sites in the sclera for bleeding and gaping.
(b) Post-operative positioning. The head must be positioned so that the gas, air or oil is lying against the hole/detachment. If a macular hole has been repaired it is especially important that the patient is positioned face down for the majority of time for ten days to two weeks after surgery. The patient can have five minutes' 'relief' from positioning every hour.

### 12.6.2   Central retinal artery occlusion

Central retinal artery occlusion is considered an ophthalmic emergency because instituting treatment within 2 hours of occurrence may restore the vision which would otherwise be permanently lost. This condition occurs suddenly, without warning, causing painless loss of vision. It is rare, usually only affecting one eye. It is caused by an embolus or thrombus due to arteriosclerosis, mitral stenosis, carotid insufficiency or temporal arteritis and as a complication of thyroid eye disease.

**Signs**

- The eye will look white.
- Visual acuity will be reduced to count fingers, hand movements or perception of light only.
- The fundus looks pale due to oedema obliterating the normal red reflex. The macula stands out as a 'cherry red spot', this area being

unaffected by the oedema as the retina here is thinner (see Section 12.1.2) and no blood vessels cross it. The red reflex from the underlying choroid can therefore be seen. The retinal arteries are small, containing segmented columns of blood called 'cattle tracking'. The retinal veins appear normal.

## Patient's needs

- Prompt medical attention for diagnosis to be made and treatment commenced.
- Investigation into the cause, and relevant treatment given if necessary.

## Nursing priorities

- Inform the medical staff immediately of the patient's visual acuity and sudden onset of symptoms.
- Prepare equipment for treatment (see below).

## Nursing action

- Instil prescribed mydriatic for ophthalmoscopic examination of the retina, so that the diagnosis can be established.
- Prepare the patient and the equipment that the doctor may require to try to restore vision. The following methods can be employed, the aim of the treatment being to dislodge the embolus or thrombus or increase the oxygen supply to the retina:
  (a)  an anterior chamber paracentesis – a needle is introduced into the anterior chamber to reduce the intra-ocular pressure suddenly;
  (b)  give 500 mg acetazolamide intravenously to reduce the intra-ocular pressure;
  (c)  massage over the globe;
  (d)  give 100% oxygen;
  (e)  ask the patient to blow into a paper bag to raise the carbon dioxide levels in the blood, which, in turn, will stimulate more oxygen to be produced;
  (f)  give a vasodilator, e.g. talazoline hydrochloride (Priscol).
    The nurse should not institute any of these measures without instructions from the doctor, as the diagnosis of sudden visual loss must be differentiated from that of a retinal detachment (see Section 12.6.1), temporal arteritis (see Section 16.5) or central retinal vein occlusion (see Section 12.6.3).
- Check blood pressure and test a specimen of urine.

If sight is not restored by any of these methods, there is no other treatment available. If sight is already poor in the other eye, the patient will need help and advice from the social services department (see Section 1.3).

### 12.6.3   Central retinal vein occlusion

Central retinal vein occlusion is a more common occurrence than retinal artery occlusion. It also affects one eye, the visual loss being sudden but usually less devastating. It is caused by hypertension, diabetes mellitus, arteriosclerosis, glaucoma and thyroid eye disease.

### Signs

- The eye will be white.
- The visual acuity will have dropped to 6/36 or less.
- The fundus will be red and swollen, with dilated and tortuous veins. Retinal haemorrhages will be present.

### Patient's needs

- Prompt medical attention so that a diagnosis can be made and treatment commenced.
- Investigation into the cause, and appropriate treatment given if necessary.

### Nursing priority

- Inform medical staff immediately of the patient's visual acuity and history of sudden onset.

### Nursing action

- Instil the prescribed mydriatic so that the fundus can be examined and a diagnosis made.
- Measure blood pressure and test a specimen of urine.
- Ensure the patient understands the instructions for the investigations.
- Ensure he understands the treatment, which may be one of the following:
  (a)   oral steroids;
  (b)   dipyridamole and aspirin to prevent the 'stickiness' of the platelets;
  (c)   photocoagulation or laser treatment to coagulate bleeding retinal vessels.

### Prognosis

Vision may recover spontaneously over several weeks or it may remain unchanged.

**Complications**

- Vitreous haemorrhage (see Section 12.9.3) from new blood vessels growing in the ischaemic retina which bleed. This could cause a retinal detachment.
- Thrombotic glaucoma (see Section 10.7.3). Neovascularisation from the ischaemic retina occurs in the iris and anterior chamber angle, blocking the drainage angle.
- Atrophy of the retina and optic nerve from ischaemia of these structures (see Section 12.8.3).
- Cystoid macular oedema (see Section 12.7.3).

### 12.6.4   Retinal haemorrhage

Retinal haemorrhage can occur in any layer of the retina, appearing as flame-shaped areas or as round blots. It can collect in the pre-retinal space between the retina and the vitreous.

**Causes**

- Vascular conditions, e.g. arteriosclerosis and hypertension (see Section 12.6.5).
- Blood diseases such as anaemia, leukaemia and sickle-cell anaemia.
- Trauma.
- Retinopathies due to diabetes, hypertension, nephritis and toxaemia of pregnancy (see below).

The treatment is that of the cause and bed rest to settle the haemorrhage. Vitrectomy may be required (see Section 12.6.1).

### 12.6.5   Retinopathies

Retinopathies are caused by diabetes mellitus, hypertension, renal disease and toxaemia of pregnancy. The result is a combination of retinal degeneration and inflammation.

### (1)  Diabetic retinopathy

Diabetic retinopathy is the leading cause of blindness in the western world in the under 65-year-olds. Diabetes, being essentially a vascular disease, affects the blood vessels of the retina. Until recently it was thought that diabetic retinopathy occurred after 20 years or so regardless of the diabetic control. Recent research (The Diabetes Control and Complications Trial Research Group 1995) indicates strongly that good control does prevent ocular and other diabetic complications. Puberty adversely affects the onset and subsequent development of retinopathy (Jose *et al.* 1994).

There are five stages of diabetic retinopathy:

- background retinopathy;
- maculopathy;
- pre-proliferative retinopathy;
- proliferative retinopathy;
- advanced retinopathy.

### Background retinopathy

Background retinopathy occurs in most diabetics about 20 years after the onset of the disease and therefore can affect all age groups from late teens onwards. It usually gives no symptoms to the patient until the macula is involved with resulting impairment of central vision. The patient may complain of glare due to the light rays being scattered by the oedematous retina.

### Signs

- The fundus has a typical picture of dots, blots and hard waxy exudates. The dots are micro-aneurysms. The blots are small haemorrhages. The hard waxy exudates are leakages of lipids from the haemorrhaging blood vessels. A ring of exudates around the macula suggests maculopathy (see below).

### Patient's needs

- Annual medical ophthalmic check-ups to assess the degree of retinopathy.
- Control of cholesterol levels by giving clofibrate tablets 500 mg three times a day.
- The patient may require advice on his treatment and diet from a diabetic clinic.

### Nursing action

- Care for the patient in the outpatient department when attending for check-ups.

### Maculopathy

Maculopathy is the main cause of visual impairment in non-insulin dependent diabetics. There are four types:

(1)  Focal/exudative. This can be treated by laser.

(2)  Cystoid/diffuse. This is difficult to treat by laser.
(3)  Ischaemic. Cannot be treated.
(4)  Mixed. Can be treated by laser.

*Patient's needs*

- Diagnosis of which type of maculopathy is present.
- Treatment with the argon laser as appropriate.
- Relief from central visual impairment.

*Nursing action*

- Prepare the patient for fundal fluorescein angiography (see Section 3.2.19).
- Prepare the patient for laser treatment (see Section 3.2.20). Laser treatment seals the leaking blood vessels around the macula, thereby reducing the production of hard exudates. The laser beam is directed at the macula but must avoid the fovea itself, as loss of central vision would result if this was hit by the beam.

### Pre-proliferative retinopathy

Pre-proliferative retinopathy may develop in eyes with background retinopathy only.

*Signs*

The retina is ischaemic which causes:

- cotton wool spots – ischaemic nerve fibre layer;
- dilation, beading, looping of blood vessels;
- arteriole narrowing;
- large dark blot haemorrhages.

There is no specific treatment unless the eye is the only seeing eye, in which case laser treatment is applied.

There are no symptoms but the patient's eyes need careful observation as they are prone to develop proliferative retinopathy.

### Proliferative retinopathy

This is the main cause of visual impairment in insulin dependent diabetics. It occurs sooner, after diagnosis of the disease, in non-insulin dependent diabetics, possibly because the disease has gone on for longer undetected. The body's natural response to the ischaemic retina is to liberate a vasoprolific factor which stimulates the formation of new blood vessels to try to overcome the lack of oxygen to the structures involved. The problem with newly formed blood vessels is that they are very fragile and bleed easily. In proliferative retinopathy these blood vessels grow into the vitreous and they bleed, causing vitreous haemorrhage. Eventually traction bands of fibrous tissue form which pull on the retina causing a retinal detachment. These new vessels can be seen easily on ophthalmoscopy and angiography.

The aim of the treatment is to prevent the neovascularisation occurring. The laser beam is applied to the retina. Dead retina will not encourage new vessel growth. Thus the retina is peppered with small areas of scotomas from laser treatment. These scotomas appear to cause little visual impairment to the patient. Vitrectomy will remove the haemorrhage. Vitrectomy will also remove the scaffold that the new vessels grow into.

*Patient's needs*

- Treatment of proliferative retinopathy by the laser to prevent further deterioration.
- Treatment of the vitreous haemorrhage.
- Guidance around the hospital if visual acuity is poor.

*Nursing action*

- Prepare the patient for laser treatment (see Section 3.2.20).
- Admit the patient to hospital and prepare for vitrectomy (see Section 12.6.1).
- Assist the severely visually handicapped patient.

**Advanced retinopathy**

This is the end result of uncontrolled proliferative retinopathy and results in blindness.

*Signs*

- Persistent vitreous haemorrhage.
- Retinal detachment.
- 'Burnt out stage' when no new vessels are stimulated to grow because the retina has become anorexic due to there being more fibrous than vascular tissue.
- Neovascular or thrombotic glaucoma due to new vessels growing in the anterior chamber angle obstructing the outflow of aqueous.

*Patient's needs*

- Vitrectomy if not performed previously.
- Treatment of neovascular glaucoma.
- Management of visual impairment.

*Nursing action*

- Prepare the patient for vitrectomy (see Section 12.6.1).
- Assist in the treatment of glaucoma.
- Instruct the patient to instil beta-blockers, e.g. Betoptic, twice a day and take acetazolamide 250 mg 4 times a day.
- Prepare the patient for laser treatment to new vessels in angle and/or for trabeculoplasty (see 'Laser treatment' in Section 10.7.2).
- Prepare the patient for trabeculectomy (see 'surgical treatment' in Section 10.7.2) or insertion of a filtering tube, e.g. Molteno, if above measures have failed.
- Inform the patient about services available and refer to social worker and low visual aid clinic as appropriate.

**(2) Hypertensive retinopathy** (including renal disease and toxaemia of pregnancy)

Hypertensive retinopathy is caused by primary hypertension and hypertension secondary to renal disease and toxaemia of pregnancy. Patients usually have no symptoms until the haemorrhages and exudates affect the macula with resulting central field involvement.

There are four stages, graded according to their severity.

*Grade I.* There is generalised arterial constriction which gives the fundal picture of 'silver' or 'copper wiring' due to increased light reflex from the thickened arterial walls.

*Grade II.* There is arteriovenous 'nipping' due to arteriosclerosis. The thickened arterial wall obscures the vein lying beneath it.

*Grade III.* In grade III haemorrhages and exudates appear. Flame-shaped haemorrhages follow the nerve fibres and are superficial. Round haemorrhages lie deeper in the retinal layers. Exudates are not in fact exudates as such but are white 'fluffy' areas of infarcted nerve fibres due to ischaemia.

*Grade IV.* All the above signs are present plus papilloedema. Renal failure will probably have occurred and vision is grossly impaired. Characteristically in renal retinopathy there is a well-defined star appearance of exudates at the macula.

**Patient's needs**

- Regular ophthalmic check-ups including fundal fluorescein angiography to document any changes in the retinal blood vessels.

- Treatment of the underlying cause. Referral to a physician may be necessary. If the toxaemia of pregnancy is severe, the pregnancy may need to be terminated to save the mother's sight and life.

*Nursing action*

- Assist the patient in the outpatient department.
- Measure blood pressure and test urine specimen.
- Prepare the patient for a fundal fluorescein angiography (see Section 3.2.19).

*Prognosis*

If the underlying cause is kept under control, visual prognosis is fairly good. Once the macular area becomes involved vision deteriorates. A severe retinopathy results in poor visual acuity and an accompanying poor prognosis. A complication of toxaemic retinopathy is a retinal detachment (see Section 12.6.1).

### 12.6.6   Retinal degenerations

Degenerations of the retina occur around its periphery. Some are significant in that they may cause retinal detachment (see Section 12.6.1). These are lattice and snail-track degeneration and acquired retinoschisis. Other degenerations, such as snowflake, paving stone and honeycomb, are insignificant causing no ophthalmic complication.

### Retinitis pigmentosa

Retinitis pigmentosa is a hereditary degeneration of the retinal nerve cells affecting 1 in 2500. The heredity is variable, resulting in varying degrees of severity. The autosomal and X-linked recessive forms are severe with symptoms starting in teenage years. The autosomal dominant form is less severe with symptoms occurring in later adult life. The rods are slowly destroyed, initially affecting the peripheral retina causing night blindness. Eventually the whole retina is affected when tunnel vision results.

An electroretinogram is performed to diagnose the condition. Later colour vision is affected. Eventually even the macula may be involved, causing total blindness. Cataracts may develop.

On ophthalmoscopy, the retina is peppered with black pigment. There is no known treatment. Management is aimed at improving visual impairment with low visual aids, pinhole spectacles and eye shields.

Couples should receive genetic counselling before starting a family if one of them is affected.

### Retinopathy of prematurity

The retinal blood vessels' development is not complete until the month after birth. Therefore a baby born prematurely will have an incompletely developed retinal blood supply. If the baby is given a high concentration of oxygen in an incubator, the stimulus for the continuing development of the retinal vessels is withdrawn. When the baby is removed from the oxygen supply, the retina is receiving insufficient oxygen and it becomes anoxic, resulting in proliferation of new vessels.

Although the oxygen now delivered to incubators is monitored closely, and must continue to be so, the condition is still occurring. It is thought to be due more to the prematurity or low birth weight of the baby than to the concentration of oxygen (Duker & Tolentino 1991). O'Connor and Glasper (1995) suggest it is a multifactoral condition.

There are five stages of the disease. Stages 1 and 2 generally regress without treatment. The other stages are treated by laser to decrease the proliferation. Visual prognosis tends to be poor. Screening of premature and low birth weight babies is essential at approximately 6 to 9 weeks after birth.

### 12.6.7   Retinal tumour: Retinoblastoma

A retinoblastoma is a retinal tumour occurring in children under the age of 5 years. It is very rare but highly malignant, occurring in 1 in 20 000 live births. It usually only affects one eye, but in 30% of cases is bilateral, both growths being primary tumours. There may be a family history of retinoblastoma.

### Signs

- A white pupil is noted, the tumour showing through the pupil instead of the normal red choroidal reflex. A white pupil may also be a sign of a cataract.
- The child may have a squint because he will not be using the affected eye for seeing and it will deviate inwards.

### Treatment

The eye will be enucleated (see Chapter 15), unless the tumour is small, in which case photocoagulation, cryotherapy, laser or radiotherapy treatment will be used, preserving the eye and maybe some sight. External beam radiation providing a lens sparing technique results in less damage to the eye than whole eye radiation (Toma *et al.* 1995). If the child presents with bilateral tumours, the sight of one eye will be preserved as far as possible without endangering the child's life. The eye with the smallest tumour will be treated by one of the methods mentioned.

Careful watch must be kept on an unaffected fellow eye. If a tumour occurs in it, it must be treated promptly as above to destroy the tumour and preserve as much sight as possible.

Siblings must be checked for the presence of a retinoblastoma and children of surviving sufferers must be examined at birth and observed until the age of 5 years.

### Prognosis

The earlier the diagnosis is made and treatment instituted, the higher the chance of preventing metastases. An untreated tumour spreads within the eye, causing it to become glaucomatous. From the eye malignant cells track back into the orbit and brain via the optic nerve and can metastasise into the liver and elsewhere in the body. A late diagnosis will result in a poorer prognosis for the child's life.

### 12.6.8   Cytomegalovirus retinitis

Cytomegalovirus (CMV) is a common member of the herpes virus family, usually remaining dormant unless the person is immunocompromised. Cytomegalovirus retinitis is the commonest opportunistic infection in people with AIDS, affecting 20–30% of sufferers (Engstrom & Holland 1995). As it is a progressive disease it can result in severe visual impairment. Recurrence of the disease heralds a particularly poor visual prognosis.

### Signs

- Retinal haemorrhages and exudates are present which progress to become necrotic eventually involving the optic disc. Retinal detachment can occur as can cataracts.

### Patient's needs

- Diagnosis of the disease.
- Medical or surgical treatment as appropriate.
- Professional counselling/referral if diagnosis of AIDS is made in the ophthalmic department.

### Nursing action

- Assist in diagnostic tests: ophthalmoscopy, fundal photography.
- Explain the different treatment modalities;

(a)  *Ganciclovir* (dihydroxypropoxymethyl guanine (DHPG))
     Induction: 5 mg/kg body weight intravenously twice a day for
     two to three weeks.
     Maintenance: single daily dose of 5 mg/kg body weight intra-
     venously every day
     **OR** 6 mg/kg body weight intravenously for five days a week
     **OR** 3 g per day oral Ganciclovir.
(b)  *Foscarnet* (trisodium phosphonoformate)
     Induction: 60 mg/kg body weight three times a day for two to
     three weeks
     Maintenance: 90–120 mg/kg body weight intravenously daily
     indefinitely.

Maintenance treatment has to be given indefinitely as the virus lies
dormant. Despite maintenance, recurrences are common.

Ganciclovir and Foscarnet treat the CMV retinitis but have no effect
on the AIDS itself. Drugs that treat the AIDS, e.g. AZT, cannot be given
concurrently with Ganciclovir as the combined drugs are too toxic to
bone marrow. Drugs similar to AZT are on trial that cause less bone
marrow toxicity.

Ganciclovir implants in the vitreous are being tried (Martin *et al.*
1994).

- Prepare the patient for retinal detachment surgery/vitrectomy (see
  Section 12.6.1).
- Refer the patient to counselling/AIDS service as appropriate.
- Employ cross-infection procedures according to local policies. It must
  be remembered that the HIV virus is very weak and does not survive
  outside the body. Although it has been isolated in tears, large quan-
  tities are required for transmission of the virus.

**Prognosis**

Patients being treated for CMV retinitis in one eye rarely get it in the
fellow eye (Jabs *et al.* 1989), whereas untreated patients have an incidence
of 60% occurrence in the fellow eye. Thus if one eye is blind from CMV
retinitis, treatment will continue to protect the other eye.

## 12.7   CONDITIONS OF THE MACULA

### 12.7.1   Age-related macular degeneration

Age-related macular degeneration is a bilateral condition affecting the
cones in the macular region, in old age. It is thought that there might be a
hereditary element and that myopia may be a predisposing factor. There
is gradual loss of central vision, but peripheral vision is retained so that
the patient will always be able to retain his 'navigational' vision. The loss

of central vision causes much distress to the patients. They are unable to recognise people because they cannot see their faces clearly, they cannot see the bus numbers, sign for their pensions, watch television clearly or read. They need continual reassurance that they will not go completely blind.

## Signs

- Pigment disturbance at the fovea spreads to the rest of the macula.
- Drusen – small yellow colloid deposits under the pigment epithelium – may precede the pigmental disturbance.
- Subretinal haemorrhages may occur. The degenerative process causes fragile new blood vessels to form. This condition is called age-related *disciform macular degeneration* and a more rapid loss of vision occurs. Laser treatment can be given for this type of degeneration, but there is no treatment if disciform degeneration has not occurred.

## Patient's needs

- Investigations into type of degeneration.
- Laser treatment if applicable.
- Low visual aids to improve vision.

## Nursing action

- Prepare the patients for fundal fluorescein angiography (see Section 3.2.19).
- Prepare the patient for laser treatment (see Section 3.2.20).
- Assist the patient with explanations and demonstrations in the aids available. These include low visual aids which are obtained from the optician and which may be one or more of the following, depending on the individual's needs:
  (a) magnifying glasses – these can be hand-held in varying shapes and sizes or made with stands to sit on the page and be moved along the line of print;
  (b) telescopic lenses – these lenses are attached to spectacles and the item to be read must be held close to the eye. This takes time to become accustomed to and can prove quite awkward for the patient. Some telescopes are illuminated with a battery;
  (c) a good light from an anglepoise-type lamp positioned correctly over the shoulder can make a lot of difference to central vision;
  (d) special aids are available to assist in signing pension books, etc. These are cardboard cutouts which can be placed over the area to be written on, guiding the patient to sign in the correct place;
  (e) magnification using computer screens may be useful.

Remember to keep reassuring the patient that peripheral navigation vision will not be lost. He may wish to be registered as blind or partially sighted (see Section 1.2).

### 12.7.2   Central serous retinopathy

Central serous retinopathy is a maculopathy affecting a younger age group than age-related macular degeneration. The cause is unknown and occurs in the 25–40 years age group, affecting men more than women. The sufferers tend to have an anxious disposition. The patients complain of a sudden painless loss of central vision, for example down to 6/18 with a central blur. The macula is elevated with a diagnostic light reflex around the macula.

The patient will be asked to read the Amsler grid to assess the size and position of the central blur. A fundal fluorescein angiogram (see Section 3.2.19) will highlight the leaking of serous fluid from the choriocapillaries through the defect in the pigment epithelium. Laser treatment can be applied to seal the leaking vessels. The condition usually resolves itself within 2–4 months.

### 12.7.3   Cystoid macular oedema/degeneration

Cystoid macular oedema/degeneration is a rare condition causing loss of central vision. The oedema results from leakages of fluid from the retinal capillaries which infiltrate the retinal layers around the macula. It occurs gradually and can be caused by diabetic retinopathy, retinal vein occlusion, uveitis and following intra-ocular surgery when the exact causative mechanism is unknown.

A fundal fluorescein angiogram shows the leaking vessels forming a petal appearance around the macula. The condition usually regresses spontaneously but there may be permanent visual loss, especially following cataract extraction. Patients who experience slow visual deterioration following intra-ocular surgery may have this condition.

## 12.8   CONDITIONS OF THE OPTIC NERVE

### 12.8.1   Optic neuritis

Optic neuritis is an inflammation, degeneration or demyelinisation of the optic nerve at the optic disc, causing sudden loss of vision.

**Causes**

• Demyelinising diseases such as multiple sclerosis.

- Systemic infections. Viral infections such as poliomyelitis, influenza, mumps and measles.
- Lebers disease is a hereditary inflammation of the optic nerve affecting men aged between 20 and 30 years. Vision is not totally lost but there is no known treatment.
- Local extension of inflammatory disease such as sinusitis, meningitis, orbital cellulitis.
- Toxic amblyopia is caused by a high intake of tobacco, alcohol, quinine and chloroquine.
- No cause may be discovered.

### Signs

- The optic disc is pale and oedematous with blurred disc margins.
- The large retinal veins are distended.

### Patient's needs

- Diagnosis of the cause of the optic neuritis.
- Institution of treatment.

### Nursing priority

- Inform the medical staff of the patient's sudden loss of vision.

### Nursing action

- Record blood pressure and test a specimen of urine.
- Instil prescribed mydriatic for ophthalmoscopic examination.
- Ensure the patient understands the blood tests and X-rays necessary to determine the cause.

### Treatment

- The underlying cause must be treated if possible. Toxic amblyopia is treated by total abstinence of the offending toxin. Patients receiving chloroquine as treatment for rheumatoid arthritis or systemic lupus erythematosus must have regular ophthalmic examinations.
- Systemic steroids.

### Prognosis

The visual loss is usually maximal within several days of onset. It will then begin to improve 2–3 weeks afterwards and a gradual recovery occurs over several months. Recurrent attacks can cause permanent damage eventually.

## 12.8.2    Retrobulbar neuritis

Retrobulbar neuritis is inflammation of the optic nerve occurring behind the optic disc. This means that changes in the nerve cannot be seen with the ophthalmoscope. The patient's vision suddenly diminishes. It has been said that retrobulbar neuritis is a condition where the patient sees nothing out of the eye and the doctor sees nothing (abnormal) in the eye.

The causes are similar to those of optic neuritis. The treatment is that of the cause plus systemic and maybe retrobulbar steroids.

## 12.8.3    Optic nerve atrophy

Atrophy of the optic nerve can result from any of a number of causes:

- vascular – central retinal artery and vein occlusion;
- degeneration and resulting atrophy from retinal diseases, such as retinitis pigmentosa, and systemic diseases, such as multiple sclerosis;
- papilloedema;
- optic and retrobulbar neuritis;
- pressure on the optic nerve from aneurysms, glaucoma, tumours and orbital disease;
- toxic conditions, such as toxic amblyopia;
- metabolic disease, such as diabetes mellitus;
- trauma.

The signs of optic atrophy are a pale optic disc and loss of pupillary reaction to light.

The visual loss is gradual resulting in varying degrees from complete blindness to scotomas, depending on the cause. The cause must be elicited so that it can be treated.

The prognosis is usually poor. Optic atrophy caused by pressure may improve once the pressure has been relieved.

## 12.9    CONDITIONS OF THE VITREOUS

### 12.9.1    Vitreous floaters

Vitreous floaters are small opacities in the vitreous which can stimulate the retina by casting a shadow on it. The mind projects the corresponding dark form onto the appropriate field of vision. Most people experience a mild degree of vitreous floaters. When looking at a uniform background they will see minute specks in their field of vision. As long as these specks move with eye movement they are not potentially dangerous.

However, an increase in the number of floaters occurs as one grows older and the vitreous gel degenerates, a condition known as syneresis.

Myopes are also prone to an increase in the number of their floaters. There is no treatment and people often learn to live with their 'friends'.

Vitreous floaters become significant in the following circumstances.

- A sudden onset of 'cobweb' or 'spider' in the vision indicates that the vitreous attachment at the optic disc has become detached, resulting in a vitreous detachment (see Section 12.9.3).
- Flashes of light indicate that the liquefied vitreous, swirling around on eye movement, is putting traction on the retina. This could progress to a retinal detachment.
- A sudden crop of black floaters indicates the presence of a retinal tear with an associated vitreous haemorrhage. This may progress to a vitreous detachment followed by a retinal detachment.

Thus it can be seen that vitreous floaters may indicate further vitreous and retinal conditions.

### 12.9.2   Posterior vitreous detachment

Posterior vitreous detachment occurs with the degeneration of the vitreous. The vitreous detaches from its attachment around the optic disc. A 'spider's web' or 'cobweb' is noticed in the vision and a sudden increase in vitreous floaters occurs. Flashing lights may also be seen as the detaching vitreous stimulates the rods and cones.

Vitreous detachment may cause vitreous haemorrhage, retinal tears and retinal detachment and should be investigated.

Patients are often very concerned about these symptoms. Information about this condition should be given to them (see Advice Sheet No. 6).

### 12.9.3   Vitreous haemorrhage

Vitreous haemorrhage may vary in degree from minimal bleeding, in which case the patient notices a few more floaters, to a massive bleed obscuring sight suddenly so the patient can only see light.

### Causes

- Trauma.
- Vascular disorders such as hypertension, leukaemia, neovascularisation especially in diabetic retinopathy, and following a central retinal vein occlusion.
- Vitreous detachment.

---

**ADVICE SHEET No. 6**
**Eye Casualty Department**

# POSTERIOR VITREOUS DETACHMENT

**What is a posterior vitreous detachment?**

Normally most of the eye is full of a jelly-like substance, the technical term for which is vitreous. In early life this is loosely adherent to the surface of the retina, the innermost layer of the eye formed of nerve cells and fibres. In middle age (or earlier in short-sighted people) the vitreous jelly may liquify and pull away from the retina causing flashing lights and large floating spots, often spidery in shape. These changes can occur quite quickly.

**Will it affect my vision?**

The floaters and cobwebs are irritating but harmless. Although they may not go away, they tend to become less irritating with time as the brain gets used to them.

Very rarely the pulling of the jelly on the retina produces a retinal tear which may cause a serious condition called retinal detachment. This may cause a large shower of new floaters across the vision and a 'curtain' of missing vision at the edge of your vision.

Your doctor has performed a very thorough examination of your eye and has found no evidence of this.

**What can be done?**

Unfortunately, nothing can be done about the floaters although they become less irritating with time.

If things change, and you develop any of the following you should return to the Casualty Department to be seen again.

(1)   A sudden 'shower' of new floaters.
(2)   New flashing or growing lights in the corner of your vision.
(3)   A 'curtain' of missing vision.

## Signs

The fundal picture will vary according to the size of the haemorrhage, from small opacities floating in the vitreous to a total haemorrhage obscuring the fundus.

**Patient's needs**

- Diagnosis of cause of haemorrhage in order that treatment can be instituted.
- Bed rest to assist absorption of haemorrhage.
- Preparation for vitrectomy.

**Nursing action**

- If visual loss has occurred suddenly, the medical staff should be informed immediately.
- Instil prescribed mydriatic drops for ophthalmoscopy.
- Admit the patient to the ward if the haemorrhage is severe enough to warrant bed rest in hospital.
- Give pre-operative care if vitrectomy is to be performed.
- If the patient is not to be admitted, ensure that he understands the importance of resting at home.
- Give post-vitrectomy care.

# 13 The Extra-ocular Muscles

## 13.1 INTRODUCTION

There are six extra-ocular muscles which move the eye in the directions of gaze. There are four rectus muscles and two oblique muscles (Fig. 13.1).

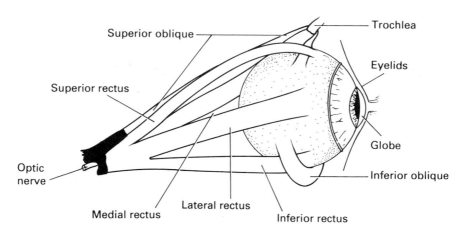

**Fig. 13.1** Diagram to show the position of the extra-ocular muscles.

(1) *The superior rectus muscle*
    Origin        – the annulus of Zinn, a tendonous ring situated around the apex of the orbit.
    Insertion     – superior sclera 7.5 mm from the limbus.
    Nerve supply  – oculomotor nerve.
    Action        – to elevate the eye.
(2) *The inferior rectus muscle*
    Origin        – the annulus of Zinn.
    Insertion     – inferior sclera 6.5 mm from the limbus.
    Nerve supply  – oculomotor nerve.
    Action        – to depress the eye.

(3)  *The medial rectus muscle*
    Origin              – the annulus of Zinn.
    Insertion          – medial sclera 5.5 mm from the limbus.
    Nerve supply – oculomotor nerve.
    Action             – to adduct the eye.

(4)  *The lateral rectus muscle*
    Origin              – the annulus of Zinn.
    Insertion          – lateral sclera 7 mm from the limbus.
    Nerve supply – abducens nerve.
    Action             – to abduct the eye.

(5)  *The superior oblique muscle*
    Origin              – the annulus of Zinn.
    Insertion          – superior outer sclera, having passed through the trochlea, a small 'pulley' situated on the medial aspect of the frontal bone (Fig. 13.1). The superior oblique muscle lies inferior to the superior rectus muscle.
    Nerve supply – trochlear nerve.
    Action             – to depress the eye.

(6)  *The inferior oblique muscle*
    Origin              – the medial aspect of the maxillary bone.
    Insertion          – posterior lateral sclera lying inferior to rectus muscle.
    Nerve supply – oculomotor nerve.
    Action             – to elevate the eye.

### 13.1.1  Blood supply

Muscular branches of the ophthalmic artery and vein are responsible for supply and drainage of blood.

## 13.2  EYE MOVEMENTS

Both eyes must move together in a coordinated manner. In order for this to occur each extra-ocular muscle is paired with a muscle in the opposite eye. These pairs of muscles are known as *synergistic* or *'yoke'* muscles. For example, to look to the right, the right eye looks outwards, i.e. abducts, while the left eye looks inwards, i.e. adducts. The right lateral rectus muscle abducts the right eye, while the left medial rectus muscle adducts the left eye. These two muscles work together to cause the eyes to look to the right. The right lateral rectus muscle and the left medial rectus muscle are therefore 'yoke' muscles.

## 13.2.1    Nine positions of gaze

To look directly upwards and downwards, two pairs of yoke muscles are required to contract. In the other positions, only one pair of yoke muscles is needed.

| *Position of gaze* | *Yoke muscles* |
|---|---|
| (1)  Straight ahead – the primary position of gaze when all the muscles are contracting to maintain the eye in this position. | |
| (2)  Upwards to the right | Right superior rectus <br> Left inferior oblique |
| (3)  To the right | Right lateral rectus <br> Left medial rectus |
| (4)  Downwards to the right | Right inferior rectus <br> Left superior oblique |
| (5)  Downwards to the left | Left inferior rectus <br> Right superior oblique |
| (6)  To the left | Left lateral rectus <br> Right medial rectus |
| (7)  Upwards to the left | Left superior rectus <br> Right inferior oblique |
| (8)  Direct elevation | Right superior rectus <br> Left inferior oblique <br> *and* <br> Left superior rectus <br> Right inferior oblique |
| (9)  Direct depression | Right inferior rectus <br> Left superior oblique <br> *and* <br> Left inferior rectus <br> Right superior oblique |

Convergence is the position of the eyes when looking at something close. In this case both medial recti contract to turn the eye inwards.

## 13.2.2    Antagonist muscles

When each muscle in the eye contracts, in order for the eye to move the antagonist or opposite muscle in the same eye must relax to allow the first muscle to work; for example, to look to the right, the right lateral rectus contracts and the right medial rectus must relax. In the left eye, the left medial rectus contracts while the left lateral rectus relaxes.

The antagonist muscles are:

- medial rectus and lateral rectus;
- inferior rectus and superior rectus;
- inferior oblique and superior oblique.


## 13.3   STRABISMUS OR SQUINT

Strabismus or squint is a deviation of one or either eye in an inward, outward, upward or downward direction (Fig. 13.2). There are many types of squint. Only the commonest will be described here. Orthoptists are highly trained to diagnose which muscle is involved and to treat the deviation in conjunction with ophthalmologists.

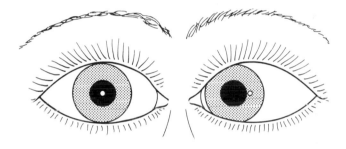

**Fig. 13.2** Left convergent squint.

A squint causes diplopia. In a child under 8 years of age, this double vision can be suppressed but an adult is unable to do this so the diplopia persists. The child suppresses the vision in the squinting eye so he no longer sees double, which is more comfortable for him. Until the age of 8 years, the visual process has not matured and if an eye is not used for any reason it may lose its ability to see. This results in reduced visual acuity, a condition called *amblyopia*. Because the visual system is not mature until the age of 8, reduced vision can be improved with treatment up to this age. Thereafter loss of visual acuity due to amblyopia will not improve. Therefore it is important that squint and any resulting amblyopia are diagnosed before the age of 8 years. This applies to all squints, whether manifest or latent. School eye tests are important to pick up poor vision before it is too late for treatment to be of help.

Normal vision with both eyes in use is termed *binocular single vision*. The images from both eyes together are seen as one visual impression by means of the fusion faculty. The aim of treatment for squint is to restore binocular single vision and prevent or reverse amblyopia.

### 13.3.1    Types of squint

Squints are either non-paralytic or paralytic.

### 13.3.2    Non-paralytic squint

Non-paralytic squint is the squint of childhood and is sometimes called a *concomitant squint*.

It can be manifest or latent, convergent or divergent, alternating or non-alternating (unilateral).

- A *manifest squint* is where one or other eye deviates from the primary or straight ahead position. It can often be an obvious squint to the observer.
- A *latent squint* is where there is a tendency for both eyes to deviate and this is not usually observed unless symptoms such as headaches or diplopia have occurred, in which case the latent squint may have become manifest.
- A *convergent squint* is a squint in which one eye turns inwards.
- A *divergent squint* is a squint in which one eye turns outwards.
- An *alternating squint* is a squint in which the eyes deviate alternately, whereas it is always the same eye which deviates in a *non-alternating squint*.

#### Causes

A non-paralytic squint occurs because there may be obstacles to the correct formation of the image falling on one retina. In other words, there is an obstruction to clear vision in the visual media which results in loss of binocular single vision.

#### *Uncorrected refractive error*

Uncorrected refractive error is the commonest cause of squint in childhood. The most usual squint is convergent, the commonest cause being hypermetropia, which causes overaccommodation and therefore over-convergence. In contrast to this, myopia can predispose to a tendency to divergence, because the eyes are already in focus to near vision without the aid of accommodation, convergence is not stimulated and divergence may result. Anisometropia (a different refraction in each eye) causes unequally clear images which can lead to a squint.

The usual pattern of events to occur, if the onset of squint is under the age of 8 years, is:

- squint leads to loss of binocular single vision;

- loss of binocular single vision results in diplopia;
- diplopia is overcome by suppression of one image;
- suppression leads to amblyopia (a reduction in visual acuity in one eye);
- the passage of time leads to loss of binocular function (the two eyes being no longer able to see one image together).

Amblyopia does not develop in an alternating squint as both eyes are used alternatively.

### Prolonged eye inactivity

Prolonged inactivity of one eye may be a dissociating factor and may enable the affected eye to deviate through disuse.

- Opacities in the media, i.e. cornea, lens, vitreous or retina, may cause squint. A cataract or retinoblastoma may present as a squint.
- Bandaging of one eye, for example following injury to the eye or a unilateral ptosis, may also cause squint.

## Examination

### History

A careful history must be taken and should include:

- family history because there may be a hereditary factor;
- age at onset which is an important factor in prognosis for reversing amblyopia and restoring binocular single vision;
- type of onset. The onset of squint may occur in one or several of the following ways:
  (a) suddenly – the squint occurs without any previous sign;
  (b) gradually – the squint appears more and more frequently and possibly increasing in size over a period of time;
  (c) intermittently, e.g. when tired, upset or unwell; the eye may be straight at other times;
  (d) constantly – the squint is present all the time;
  (e) changing in size at different times of day;
  (f) when looking in a particular position of gaze or at a particular distance;
  (g) either eye may deviate alternatively or it may always be the same eye that deviates.
  The onset may be associated with some systemic disease because the child is generally unwell.

## Visual acuity

Visual acuity will be recorded using the Snellen chart, Sheridan Gardiner Test or other tests.

## Determination of refractive error

In children a cycloplegic drop such as G. cyclopentolate is needed to prevent accommodation, which would give a false result on retinoscopy. A retinoscope directs a light beam onto the retina and movement of the retinoscope produces movement of the light beam across the retina in a particular direction. A lens is selected and held in front of the eye while continuing to move the retinoscope. A change is noted in the amount and direction of the movement of the light beam. Finally, the lens, which actually neutralises or abolishes the movement of the light beam, determines the refractive error.

## Physical examination

(1)  The presence of the following features is noted:
   •  epicanthus – if a child has broad epicanthic folds, it can give the appearance of a convergent squint, but if the cover test is negative this is called a *pseudosquint*;
   •  ptosis or other feature leading to asymmetry of the palpebral apertures;
   •  nystagmus;
   •  an abnormal head posture, which could be compensating for squint;
   •  unequal pupil sizes.
(2)  An inspection of the eyes is carried out:
   •  corneal reflections;
   •  cover test;
   •  ocular movements;
   •  measuring the angle of deviation;
   •  stereoscopic vision.
     The Photoscreener has been developed to detect squint, refractive errors and media opacities in young children without cyclopegia (Ottar *et al.* 1995).

### Corneal reflections

#### Method
A pen torch is held at $\frac{1}{3}$ m directly in front of both eyes The position of the reflection on each eye is then compared.

*Results*
The results may be:

- normal corneal reflections – symmetrical (Fig. 13.3);
- asymmetrical corneal reflections (Fig. 13.4).

An upturning eye or a downturning eye can also be detected by observing the corneal reflections (such squints are less common).

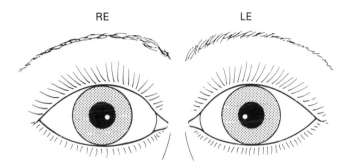

The corneal reflections are symmetrical, usually slightly nasal in each eye.

*Note:* corneal reflections may not be central, but check **symmetry**.

**Fig. 13.3** Normal corneal reflections – symmetrical.

*Cover test*

The cover test is carried out to detect the presence of a squint, and should be used in conjunction with observation of the corneal reflections.

*Method*
A penlight is held approximately $\frac{1}{3}$ m from the child. The child must be looking at the light whilst the cover test is carried out. It is important to repeat the cover test using a detailed target, e.g. a small picture on a tongue depressor, because some squints are only present when looking at detailed objects. The cover test should also be carried out at 6 m where possible because other squints are only present when looking into the distance, i.e. intermittent squints.

Cover one eye, watching for any movement of the uncovered eye, remove the cover and repeat covering the other eye and watching for any movement of the uncovered eye.

*Results*
The results may be:

- no manifest squint (Fig. 13.5);

RE                    LE

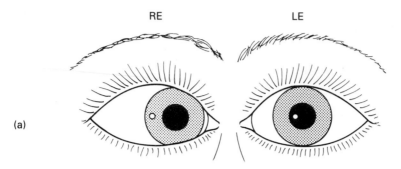

(a)

Note asymmetry of corneal reflections.

The left corneal reflection is in the normal position, i.e. slightly nasal.

The right corneal reflection is displaced temporally, because the right eye is turning inwards.

RE                    LE

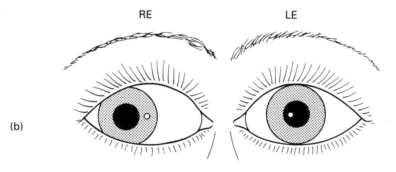

(b)

Note asymmetry of corneal reflections.

The left corneal reflection is in the normal position, i.e. slightly nasal.

The right corneal reflection is displaced nasally, because the right eye is turning outwards.

**Fig. 13.4** Asymmetrical corneal reflections. (a) Right convergent squint and (b) right divergent squint.

- manifest squint – right convergent squint (Fig. 13.6);
- manifest squint – right divergent squint (Fig. 13.7).

An intermittent convergent squint may not be present when the child is looking at a light but becomes manifest when focusing on a detailed target. Therefore it is important to check the corneal reflections and to carry out the cover test using a light *and* a detailed target.

An intermittent divergent squint may not be present for near but

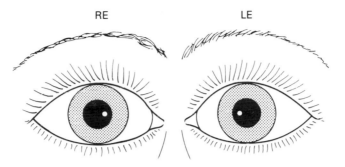

The corneal reflections are symmetrical, i.e. no manifest squint detected.

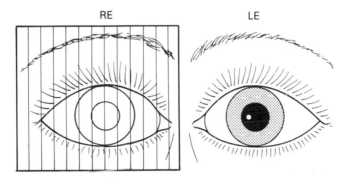

No movement of the left eye when the right eye is covered.

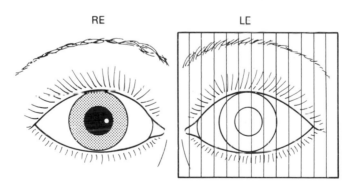

No movement of the right eye when the left eye is covered.

**Fig. 13.5** No manifest squint.

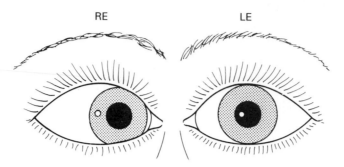

RE                                        LE

The corneal reflections are asymmetrical, showing a right convergent squint.

Confirm with cover test.

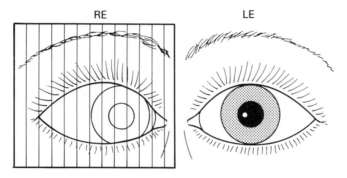

RE                                        LE

No movement of the left eye when the right eye is covered.

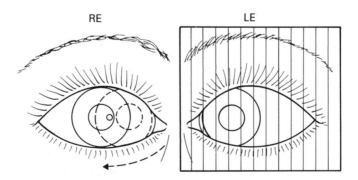

RE                                        LE

The right eye moves *out* to fix when the left eye is covered.

**Fig. 13.6** Manifest squint – right convergent squint.

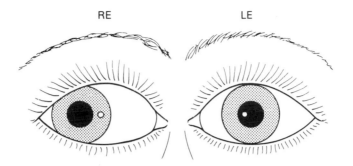

The corneal reflections are asymmetrical, showing a right divergent squint.

Confirm with cover test.

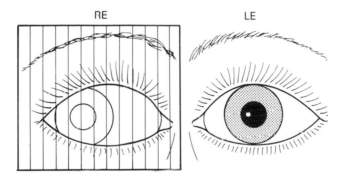

No movement of the left eye when the right eye is covered.

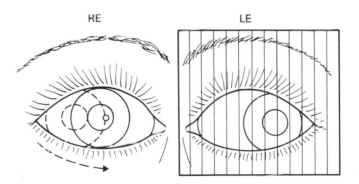

The right eye moves *in* to fix when the left eye is covered.

**Fig. 13.7** Manifest squint – right divergent squint.

becomes manifest in the distance. Therefore it is important to carry out a cover test for near *and* distance.

The cover test for a latent squint, or an alternate cover test, is where the occluder covers one eye then the other. Observation of the eye that has just been covered is noted.

## *Ocular movements*

The examiner sits in front of the patient and using a pen torch, and a toy if appropriate, observes both eyes moving in all eight positions of gaze. This will include up, down, both sides and in all four corners, always returning to the straight ahead or primary position. The patient's head must be held still. Any muscle imbalance, over actions and under actions are then noted.

## *Measuring the angle of deviation*

The angle of deviation can be measured using objective or subjective methods.

Objective methods are based on the observer neutralising the patient's deviation as it takes up fixation. Subjective measurements are where the patient tells you the position of each image from each eye on a calibrated scale of some sort.

The following methods include both objective and subjective measurements.

- *Prisms and cover test.* This is the most commonly used objective method of measuring the angle of a manifest or a latent squint.

  The measurements are performed at near ($\frac{1}{3}$m), distance (6 m) and occasionally beyond 6 m (far distance).

  Loose prisms, or a prism bar, are introduced in front of the squinting eye in a manifest squint, or in front of either eye in a latent squint, with the apex of the prism in the direction of the deviation.
- *Major amblyoscope (synoptophore).* The angle of deviation can be measured both objectively and subjectively. Slides are introduced and the measurement can be read from the scales in degrees or prism dioptres.
- *Maddox rod and Maddox wing.* The Maddox rod is used in conjunction with a light at 6 m and measures small degrees of squint. The Maddox rod is made of a series of parallel cylinders, red in colour, which convert a light image into a red line. This is placed before one eye while the patient is fixing on a light at 6 m distance with both eyes open. The eye looking through the Maddox rod sees a red line instead of a white light and the other eye sees the light as it really is. These images are too dissimilar for fusion to take place, so the eyes deviate to

the position of squint. Prisms are introduced until the light and the red line are superimposed.

The Maddox wing enables measurements of latent and small manifest deviations to be made at a near distance.

The Maddox rod and wing allow measurement of horizontal and vertical deviations. The wing also allows torsional measurements to be made.

*Stereoscopic vision*

The ability to see in 'depth' or 3D vision is the highest form of binocular sight. The main tests measuring stereo acuity in seconds of arc (the measurement of minimum disparity that gives rise to appreciation of depth) include:

(1)  Frisby test;
(2)  Wirt fly test (Titmus test);
(3)  TNO (red/green test);
(4)  Lang stereo test.

**Treatment** (see Patient Information Leaflet No. 5)

Treatment for a non-paralytic squint falls under four headings (each beginning with the letter 'O').

(1)  *Optical treatment.* Accurate refraction must be carried out and appropriate glasses ordered. This in itself might correct the squint.
(2)  *Occlusion therapy.* The visual acuity must be assessed, and if amblyopia is present, it must be reversed. This is performed by occluding the 'good' eye to encourage the amblyopic eye to work. Occlusion therapy is carried out, according to the state of amblyopia, in the following ways:
     (a)  total occlusion – the patch is placed over the 'good' eye itself;
     (b)  partial occlusion – the lens of the glasses is covered with tape or paper;
     (c)  constant occlusion – (a) or (b) used from morning till night;
     (d)  part-time occlusion – (a) or (b) used for a specified number of hours each day.
(3)  *Orthoptic exercises* are used to stimulate binocular single vision and strengthen fusion by means of binocular instruments such as the synoptophore. This instrument uses pairs of slides, one for each eye, which match together to form a picture; a bird seen with one eye and a cage seen with the other will be seen with both eyes together as a bird in a cage.

## PATIENT INFORMATION LEAFLET No. 5

# SQUINT SURGERY FOR CHILDREN

Your child has been put on the waiting list for surgery. This leaflet aims to answer questions you may have in anticipation of the operation.

**Why does my child need surgery?**

Your child has a muscle imbalance that has resulted in one of the eyes turning in, out, up or down. The consultant has now decided that he/she would benefit from an operation to correct the imbalance.

Other treatment may also be carried out in conjunction with surgery.

- *Patching*

The outcome of surgery is generally better if there is a good level of vision in the squinting eye.

- *Glasses*

If your child wears glasses, these should be worn constantly as the operation will correct the amount that the eye turns when he/she is wearing the glasses.

In a few cases, neither of the above treatments are necessary and surgery is offered to you soon after your first appointment.

**When will my child have the operation?**

He/she has been put on the waiting list. The waiting time for squint surgery varies between consultants and you should have been given an approximate waiting time when you were added to the list.

If you have not heard from the Eye Unit for a long period of time, you may telephone the admission office to ask about further waiting time. When you call, you will need to know the following:

- Hospital number.
- Consultant's name.
- The date your child's name was added to the list.

**How long will he/she be in hospital?**

All squint surgery is done as a day case. You will be sent a pre-assessment appointment for 1–2 weeks before the operation date when an orthoptist will measure the squint and the pre-assessment team will check that your child is fit for surgery. You will be expected to arrive early on the day of the operation and normally allowed home towards the end of the day.

If your child's general health changes between the pre-assessment and the operation, you must visit your doctor. If your doctor thinks that your child is not fit for surgery, you must contact the Eye Unit immediately.

▶

**PATIENT INFORMATION LEAFLET No. 5** *continued*

**Can I stay with my child?**

We encourage you to stay with your child. Please make arrangements for the care of any other children for the whole day.

**What sort of anaesthetic will it be?**

All squint surgery in children is done under a general anaesthetic. This means that your child will be asleep throughout the operation.

As your child will be having an anaesthetic you must starve him/her for 6 hours before the operation.

**What do I need to bring with me?**

- All current medicines.
- Glasses.
- Dressing gown (if you have one).
- Toiletries.
- A box of tissues.
- A note of any drug allergies.
- One cuddly toy (there are plenty of toys on the ward) and/or a comforter.
- Own special cup if one is used.

**What does the operation involve?**

Squint surgery is the repositioning of the muscles. This involves making a small incision in the tissue covering the eye which allows the surgeon to access the underlying muscles. The eyeball is NEVER removed from the socket.

**Will he/she have a pad on the eye following the operation?**

No, the eye will not be padded, as this can be distressing for your child. Immediately after the operation, you should try and stop him/her rubbing the eye.

**After the operation**

Your child will normally bounce back to normal life quite quickly. He/she should be fit enough to return to school within a week.

You will be given drops to put in for two weeks after the operation to avoid infection and inflammation.

You should avoid situations where there is a risk of getting something in their eye, e.g. the sand pit at play school.

Avoid getting the eye wet. Bathe rather than shower and be careful when you wash their hair.

Avoid swimming for four weeks after the operation.

At the pre-assessment appointment you will be given an appointment time for 1–2 weeks after the operation. It is essential that you attend this appointment.

▶

---

**PATIENT INFORMATION LEAFLET No. 5** *continued*

Glasses should continue to be worn after surgery, unless told otherwise by the doctor.

If you have any further questions about the squint surgery, do not hesitate to telephone the orthoptic department or enquire at your next appointment.

Even though your child is now on the waiting list for surgery, you must continue with the other recommended treatments and keep your orthoptic appointments.

Address:
Anytown Eye Unit
Anytown General Hospital
Any Road
Anytown
AN00 0AN

**Useful telephone numbers**

Ward ............
Casualty ............
Outpatients ............
Orthoptics ............
Admissions ............

---

(4)  *Operative measures.*
  (a)  Early surgery is performed if there is:
      (i)   potential binocular function present;
      (ii)  poor cosmetic appearance with no binocular vision.
  (b)  Surgery can be delayed if the deviation is cosmetically quite good.
  (c)  Surgery is not performed if the cosmetic appearance is good in the presence of no binocular function.

Surgery will not improve binocular vision once it has been lost. The muscles operated on in convergent and divergent squint are usually the medial and lateral recti. They may be resected (shortened) or recessed (effectively lengthened). Sometimes surgery is directed to the non-squinting eye, which worries parents and sometimes nurses! It may not matter which eye is operated on, the aim being to align one eye with the other.

### 13.3.3  Paralytic squint

A paralytic or incomitant squint is more common in adults than in children. If it occurs in a child under the age of 8 years, the child will be able to suppress the resulting double vision and the events that occur with a non-paralytic squint will follow.

Adults, however, have no capacity to suppress the vision in one eye to eliminate the diplopia. This can be distressing and can be associated with nausea and giddiness.

## Causes

A paralytic squint is caused by an abnormality in the extra-ocular muscles or their nerve supply.

### *Muscle disorders*

- Trauma, e.g. forceps delivery at birth.
- Congenital abnormality.
- Disease, e.g. exophthalmic ophthalmoplegia from:
  - (a)   thyroid eye disease;
  - (b)   myasthenia gravis;
  - (c)   neoplasm.

### *Nerve disorders*

- Trauma:
  - (a)   bruising or severing of nerves following head injury;
  - (b)   pressure on nerves from haemorrhage;
  - (c)   septic infection.
- Inflammation:
  - (a)   mastoid disease;
  - (b)   peripheral neuritis;
  - (c)   encephalitis;
  - (d)   multiple sclerosis;
  - (e)   tertiary syphilis;
  - (f)   haemorrhage;
  - (g)   thrombosis;
  - (h)   aneurysm;
  - (i)   neoplasm, e.g. pituitary tumour;
  - (j)   diabetes mellitus;
  - (k)   temporarily following cataract extraction.

## Treatment

- Orthoptic assessment to establish which muscle is affected, e.g. examination of eye movements, the Hess chart and diplopia tests.
- Referral to a neurologist or physician for investigation of the cause.
- Teach compensatory head posture, if this is applicable. The patient is taught to hold his head in the position which relieves the diplopia.
- Occlude one eye if the diplopia is intolerable.

- Give temporary Fresnel prism to join the diplopia to binocular single vision if possible.
- . Botulinum can be used to paralyse muscles and thereby straighten the eye.
- Wait 6–9 months for recovery to occur.
- If recovery does not occur after 9 months, surgery can be performed to restore binocular single vision.

### Patient's needs (non-paralytic and paralytic squint)

- Correction of squint for cosmetic reasons. (Children are especially teased at school.)
- Correction of amblyopia and restoration of binocular single vision.
- Relief of diplopia if an adult.

### Nursing action (non-paralytic and paralytic squint)

- Assist with examination in the outpatient department.
- Instil prescribed cycloplegic drops, e.g. G. cyclopentolate hydro-chloride.
- Liaise with the orthoptic department if necessary about patching and exercises, and offer teaching and encouragement to the parents and child on the use of patching.
- Give advice on occluding one eye, prisms in glasses or compensatory head posture to relieve the symptoms.
- Prepare the patient for botulinum injections.
- Admit the patient to hospital if surgery is to be performed.
- Give pre-operative care, e.g. explain reasons for possibility of surgeon operating on the 'good' eye. Warn adult patients that they may feel unwell for about a week; the reason for this is not readily understood.
- Give post-operative care.
  - (a) The eye is not usually padded post-operatively.
  - (b) There may be conjunctival injection present, including a sub-conjunctival haemorrhage.
  - (c) Instil prescribed antibiotic or steroid and antibiotic drops.
  - (d) Give analgesia intramuscularly if adjustable sutures have been employed prior to their being adjusted. This can occur any time from immediately coming round from the anaesthetic to 24 hours later. Adjustable sutures are suitable for any patient over the age of 10 years (Pratt-Johnson & Tillson 1994).
  - (e) Liaise with the orthoptic department regarding the necessity of continuing with non-surgical treatment such as wearing glasses, occlusion, etc.
- Ensure that the patient has a follow-up orthoptic appointment on discharge.

**Complications (non-paralytic and paralytic squint)**

- Stitch abscess.
- The muscle slipping away from its new position because the sutures have broken.
- Failure of the operation to result in binocular single vision when this is the expected outcome.
- Failure of the operation to give a good cosmetic result.
- Overcorrection of the squint. A convergent squint results in a consecutive divergent squint, and vice versa.

### 13.3.4   Pseudosquint

A pseudosquint is the appearance of a squint occurring in the presence of binocular single vision.

**Causes**

- Epicanthus.
- Abnormal angle alpha. This is a larger or smaller than normal angle between the optic axis and the visual axis. This angle is very similar to that of angles kappa and gamma.
- Facial asymmetry.
- Wide or narrow interpupillary distance. A wide interpupillary distance gives the appearance of divergent squint, and a narrow interpupillary distance, convergent squint.

# 14  Ophthalmic Trauma

## 14.1  INTRODUCTION

The ophthalmic nurse requires special skills of observation (see Chapter 3), history taking and the ability to care for a patient who has received trauma to the eye or its surrounding area (see Chapter 2).

Penetrating (perforating) injury and ocular burns are considered ophthalmic emergencies. Blunt trauma can result in serious ocular damage. Therefore the nurse must take an accurate history, examine the eye carefully and decide in what order of priority each patient presenting with ocular trauma needs to be placed.

A blow to the eyeball causes shock waves to pass through it, damaging many structures such as the cornea, iris, lens and retina. Blunt trauma may accompany a penetrating injury, therefore any patient presenting with a history of a forceful blow to the eye must have all ocular structures examined carefully. The importance of accurate history taking cannot be over emphasised.

It is assumed in the following text that all patients will be treated for accompanying shock if present and that this may be a priority. Where appropriate a tetanus toxoid injection must be given if the skin or ocular tissue has been cut.

## 14.2  INTRA-OCULAR FOREIGN BODY

An intra-ocular foreign body (IOFB) results when something enters the eye under force, such as fragments generated when using a hammer and chisel or a lathe. The foreign body may lodge itself in any of the structures of the eye and examination may not reveal its presence, highlighting the importance of history taking.

### 14.2.1  Patient's needs

- Thorough ocular examination to determine the extent of the injuries.
- Explanation of the extent of the injuries and the required treatment.

- Admission to hospital for removal of the IOFB.
- Post-operative and discharge care.

### 14.2.2   Nursing action

- Obtain accurate history.
- Inform medical staff.
- Prepare the patient for an X-ray to locate the IOFB.
- Prepare the patient for removal of the foreign body if one is present. If it is metallic it may be removed with a specialised magnet in the operating theatre.
- Give post-operative care, clean the eye, instil drops and give any necessary information.
- Plan discharge.

## 14.3   FRACTURE OF THE ORBIT

Fractures of the orbit occur as a result of trauma. Usually they are easily recognised by the irregularity of the outline of the orbit. A 'blow-out' fracture of the orbit occurs following trauma to the maxillary bone which fractures and the eye tends to sink down into the gap created in the bone.

### 14.3.1   Signs

- Enophthalmos.
- Inability to move the eye in all fields of gaze because the extra-ocular muscles have become trapped in the fractured bone.
- Jerky eye movement in the upward gaze because the inferior oblique muscle has been trapped.

### 14.3.2   Patient's needs

- Diagnosis of the presence of a fracture.
- Relief of symptoms of:
   (a)   decreased sensation of the skin over the maxilla;
   (b)   diplopia.
- Repair of skin laceration if present.
- Repair of fracture if severe (may not be performed for up to 6 months).
- Cleaning of any wounds present.

### 14.3.3   Nursing action

- Explain to the patient the extent of the injuries and the treatment to be carried out.

- Preparation for X-ray examination to confirm and isolate the fracture.
- Clean wound if present.
- Admit the patient to the ward if surgery is to be performed.
- Prepare the patient for the operation to free the trapped muscles and repair the fracture. A Teflon plate or orbital implant may be inserted.
- Give post-operative care:
  - (a) clean the wound;
  - (b) instil antibiotic drops.
- Plan discharge.
- Remove sutures, usually as an outpatient procedure, 5 to 7 days post-operatively.

## 14.4   TRAUMA TO THE EYELIDS

Trauma to the eyelids is a common occurrence as their function is to protect the globe. The following may occur:

- bruising;
- laceration;
- burns.

### 14.4.1   Patient's needs

- Exploration of the extent of the injuries.
- Relief of symptoms. If a subtarsal foreign body is present there will be profuse lacrimation and blepharospasm.
- Treatment of injuries.

### 14.4.2   Nursing priorities

- Inform medical staff.
- Commence irrigation if a burn has occurred.

### 14.4.3   Nursing action

- Explain to the patient the extent of the injuries received and the necessary treatment.
- Assist the doctor in examining the eye.
- Treat the injuries.
  - (a) Bruising: apply cold compress and instruct the patient how to do this.
  - (b) Laceration:
    - (i)  clean wound;
    - (ii) prepare the patient and equipment for suturing of the

laceration or apply Steristrip if superficial. The two edges of the lacerated lid must be aligned very carefully to prevent trichiasis occurring.

    (c)   Burns:
- (i)    clean area;
- (ii)   irrigate eye (see Section 3.2.12);
- (iii)  admit patient if necessary;
- (iv)  apply dressings;
- (v)   prepare the patient for skin grafting which may need to be carried out before scar tissue forms.

    (d)   Subtarsal foreign body: remove the foreign body (see Section 3.2.9).

## 14.5   TRAUMA TO THE LACRIMAL SYSTEM

Laceration of the lacrimal drainage apparatus is fairly common. If the canaliculus is torn accurate apposition of the tear ducts must be performed to prevent permanent epiphora. In children the injury is often caused by the claws of a dog as it jumps up to greet the child.

### 14.5.1  Patient's needs

- Cleaning of the wound.
- Admission to hospital if necessary.
- Repair of the laceration.
- Prophylactic antibiotic cover.

### 14.5.2  Nursing priorities

- Inform medical staff of the extent of the injuries.

### 14.5.3  Nursing action

- Clean the wound.
- Assist the doctor to examine the wound.
- Admit the patient to the ward if necessary.
- Prepare the patient for surgery to repair the laceration.
- Give post-operative care:
  - (a)   clean the wound;
  - (b)   instil antibiotic drops;
  - (c)   give oral antibiotics if prescribed;
  - (d)   remove sutures 5 to 7 days post-operatively.

## 14.6   TRAUMA TO THE CONJUNCTIVA

### 14.6.1   Subconjunctival haemorrhage

Subconjunctival haemorrhage (Fig. 14.1) can result from a penetrating or blunt trauma which causes the conjunctival blood vessels to bleed.

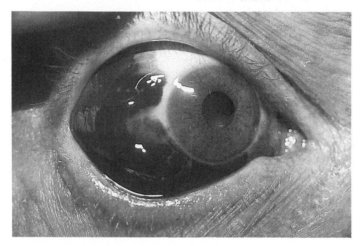

**Fig. 14.1** Subconjunctival haemorrhage.

**Patient's needs**

- Investigation into the extent of the injuries.

**Nursing action**

- Obtain accurate history.
- Examine the patient or assist the doctor. It is important to be able to visualise the scleral margin posterior to the bleed. If it is absent the bleeding may have tracked from elsewhere, typically the anterior cranial fossa, and is more serious.
- Reassure the patient that the haemorrhage will not cover the cornea thereby not affecting vision.
- Inform the patient that the blood may spread before it resolves and that it may take 2 to 3 weeks to clear completely, similar to a bruise. There is no specific treatment for the haemorrhage.

### 14.6.2   Laceration of the conjunctiva

Laceration of the conjunctiva may occur as a result of trauma to the eye. The eye must be examined to see if the underlying sclera has been involved. If there is a possibility of a foreign body having entered the eye, an X-ray must be taken to exclude or confirm this.

### Patient's needs

- Cleaning and examination of the wound and eye to discover the extent of the injuries.
- Suturing of the wound if necessary. This is not always performed.
- Prophylactic antibiotic cover.

### Nursing action

- Inform the doctor of the patient's condition.
- Assist the doctor in the examination.
- Prepare the patient and equipment for cleaning and suturing of the laceration under local anaesthetic, unless the patient is a child, when a general anaesthetic will usually be administered. Small lacerations may be left to heal without suturing.
- Apply pad following the procedure.

## 14.7 OCULAR BURNS

Ocular burns can result in patients losing their sight.

Acid substances entering the eye coagulate with the protein of the ocular surface and cease to act although damage is caused by the initial impact. Alkaline substances, such as lime found in cement and brick dust, continue to be active in the eye, destroying the superficial layers and penetrating the anterior segment of the eye. Collagenase is released by the cornea following an alkali burn and this destroys the cornea. It is therefore vitally important that the eye(s) are thoroughly cleaned of all particles of lime. Immediate washing of the eye with whatever harmless liquid is at hand is the best first aim measure that can be employed. The patient should then be transferred to an ophthalmic unit.

### 14.7.1 Patient's needs

- Irrigation of eye(s).
- Treatment of burns to the lids and skin around the eye that may have occurred.
- Reassurance and information on the extent of the injuries and treatment. Patients can be very worried about the threat of sight loss following a chemical burn.
- Pain relief.

### 14.7.2   Nursing priorities

- If a severe alkali burn has occurred, inform the doctor immediately of the patient's arrival.
- Check the pH of the conjunctival sac (normally 7.1–8.6).
- Commence irrigation of the eye(s) (see Section 3.2.12). If single-handed commence the irrigation before informing the doctor.

### 14.7.3   Nursing action

- Irrigate the eye(s) (see Section 3.2.12). Ensure all particles have been removed. It may be necessary to double evert the lid.
- Allay anxiety.
- Test visual acuity once the patient's condition allows you to.
- Institute the following treatment which will be prescribed after the eye has been examined to elicit the extent of the damage to the conjunctiva and the cornea.

### Mild burns

(a)   Instil G. homatropine 2% to 'rest' the eye and prevent uveitis.
(b)   Instil G. or Oc. chloramphenicol to prevent infection and provide lubrication.
(c)   Apply a pad to aid comfort and healing.
(d)   Give prescribed analgesia.

### Moderate to severe burns (Fig. 14.2)

(a)   Instil ascorbate drops to aid healing, intensively such as hourly initially, reducing to 2 hourly after three days.

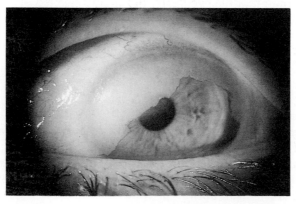

**Fig. 14.2** Lime burn.

(b)    Instil G. chloramphenicol to prevent infection.
(c)    Instil a steroid such as G. Maxidex (dexamethasone) to prevent/treat inflammation.
(d)    Instil G. homatropine 2% to 'rest' the eye and prevent/treat uveitis.

- Drugs that inhibit collagenase such as metaloproteinase inhibitors may be used.
- Apply a bandage contact lens to prevent symblephron forming (see Section 14.6.5). Rodding of the fornices may be employed.
- Apply steroid ointment to the skin around the eye if prescribed.

### 14.7.4    Other treatments

The excimer laser has been used to treat chemical burns. Keratoepithelioplasty (KEP) or cadaveric limbal cell transplantation has been successfully employed as well (Anon 1995).

### 14.7.5    Complications

#### Symblephron

Symblephron is the adhesion of the bulbar conjunctiva to the palpebral conjunctiva (Fig. 14.3). It occurs following alkaline burns to the eye when the epithelial layer of the conjunctiva is stripped off and the two areas of the conjunctiva stick together. When this occurs the fornices are lost and the eye is immobile. The lids may not be able to cover and protect the eyeball. It is therefore important to keep the fornices well lubricated and to apply a bandage contact lens to separate the two conjunctival surfaces

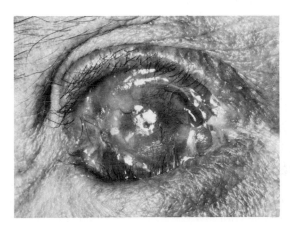

**Fig. 14.3** Symblephron.

or to rod them to break up any adhesions that might occur. This latter procedure can be painful. Nasal mucosal grafts can be performed.

### Corneal opacities

Corneal opacities occur from destruction of the layers of the cornea from the burns. Blindness may result.

### 14.7.6  Welder's flash

Welder's flash or a burn from a sun lamp or snowblindness burn the cornea if protective goggles have not been worn. Both eyes are affected and become very red and sore.

### Patient's needs

- Relief of symptoms of:
  - (a)  acute pain;
  - (b)  watering;
  - (c)  photophobia;
  - (d)  reduced vision.

  These symptoms do not become evident until about 8 hours after the incident has occurred.

### Nursing action

- Instil local anaesthetic drops.
- Institute prescribed treatment once the eye has been examined. G. fluorescein shows punctate staining over most of the cornea, especially within a central band. The treatment is with:
  - (a)  Oc. chloramphenicol immediately – once only;
  - (b)  pad and bandage if severe. Both eyes may need to be bandaged for comfort and healing.

### 14.8   TRAUMA TO THE CORNEA

### 14.8.1  Corneal foreign bodies

Many different kinds of foreign bodies can adhere to the cornea: dirt specks, sawdust, pieces of metal or rust (Fig. 14.4). Anyone working in an environment, whether at work or at home, where particles can fly into the eye, or working with a hammer and chisel, should wear protective goggles. But these do not always afford complete protection.

The eye with a corneal foreign body present may or may not be red,

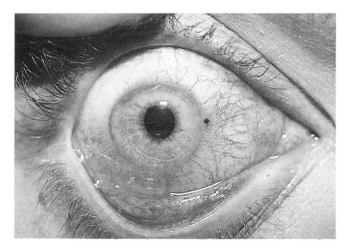

**Fig. 14.4** Metallic corneal foreign body.

depending on what the foreign body is, how long it has been in the eye and how much the patient has rubbed it.

**Patient's needs** (see Advice Sheet No. 7)

* Removal of the foreign body to relieve pain and discomfort.
* Treatment of any corneal abrasion.

**Nursing action**

* Record the visual acuity before removal of the foreign body. This is particularly important if the accident has occurred at work. It may be necessary to instil a drop of local anaesthetic into the eye before the patient can read the Snellen chart.
* Remove/assist the doctor to remove the foreign body (see Section 3.2.9).
* Apply antibiotic ointment.
* Apply a pad if necessary for patient comfort but bear in mind recent research indicating that the corneal epithelium is slower to heal under a pad (Kirkpatrick *et al.* 1993).
* If the foreign body is a piece of metal, a rust ring may be left around the abrasion resulting from the foreign body. This rust ring will need to be removed either at the first visit or the following one. A dental burr may be used for this procedure.
* Instil G. homatropine 2% to prevent the complication of uveitis occurring.
* Ensure the patient is not driving if he has an eye pad on. Although it is

---

**ADVICE SHEET No. 7**
**Eye Casualty Department**

# FOREIGN BODIES ON THE EYE

The doctor or nurse has removed a piece of foreign material (e.g. metal or wood) from the front of your eye. Although most of these injuries heal up completely, there are several things you should bear in mind:

(1)  Although the eye may be comfortable on your leaving the hospital, it may become uncomfortable again in about 30 minutes, when the anaesthetic drops wear off. Use the treatment prescribed for you.

(2)  Normally the eye should heal up and become comfortable again in about 24 hours. It is not generally necessary to see you again, but you should return after this time if the eye seems to be getting increasingly red or sore or the vision more blurred.

(3)  When necessary, protect your eyes with some form of goggles. This is essential when hammering or grinding, etc.

**Further advice and instructions**

. . . . . . . . . . . . . . . . . . . . . . . . . . . . . . . . . . . . . . . . . . . . . . . . . . . . . . . . . . . . . . . . .
. . . . . . . . . . . . . . . . . . . . . . . . . . . . . . . . . . . . . . . . . . . . . . . . . . . . . . . . . . . . . . . . .
. . . . . . . . . . . . . . . . . . . . . . . . . . . . . . . . . . . . . . . . . . . . . . . . . . . . . . . . . . . . . . . . .
. . . . . . . . . . . . . . . . . . . . . . . . . . . . . . . . . . . . . . . . . . . . . . . . . . . . . . . . . . . . . . . . .

---

not illegal to drive with one eye padded, it is not safe to do so and the patient's insurance will not be valid. Stereoscopic vision is lost and the field of vision reduced, especially if the right eye is covered. If the patient has arrived by car and there is no-one to take him home, he can be given a pad to apply at home following instructions on how to do so.

• Ensure the patient understands the need for any follow-up visit(s) required to check on healing.

## Complications

• Corneal ulceration.
• Corneal scarring.

### 14.8.2    Corneal abrasion

Corneal abrasions can result from a foreign body as seen above. Other common causes are babies' fingernails, twigs, flower stalks, pens and pencils. In fact a great variety of items can cause abrasion.

#### Patient's needs

- Relief of symptoms, which can vary in severity:
  - (a)   pain;
  - (b)   lacrimation;
  - (c)   photophobia;
  - (d)   blepharospasm;
  - (e)   reduced vision.
- Treatment of the abrasion.

#### Nursing action

- Record visual acuity. It may be necessary to instil a local anaesthetic drop first.
- Examine/assist the doctor to examine the eye. The abraded area will show up with the instillation of G. fluorescein and illumination with a blue light.
- Institute prescribed treatment:
  - (a)   if large, G. homatropine 2% will be instilled to prevent uveitis and afford some pain relief as the pupil will dilate and prevent iris spasm;
  - (b)   apply oc. chloramphenicol;
  - (c)   apply a pad or pad and bandage if the abrasion is large (see Section 3.2.4).
- Warn the patient that this condition will be painful and ensure he has adequate analgesia to take.
- Ensure the patient understands the need for any follow-up visit(s) required to check on healing. A large abrasion may take several days to heal.

#### Complications

- Corneal ulceration.
- Recurrent corneal abrasion/erosion. These can recur up to one year or longer after the initial incident. The patient on waking finds he has difficulty opening the eye and that it is painful. On examination the epithelium will have debrided again. This occurs because the epithelium is loosely adherent to Bowman's membrane. There may be an hereditary tendency to recurrent erosions. The treatment is as above. The excimer laser has been used to treat these erosions. Application of

eye ointment such as simple eye ointment or Oc. chloramphenicol at night can prevent this recurring condition.

### 14.8.3   Perforation of the cornea

Usually when the cornea perforates from injury, the iris herniates into the perforation, blocking it and causing the anterior chamber to collapse (Fig. 14.5).

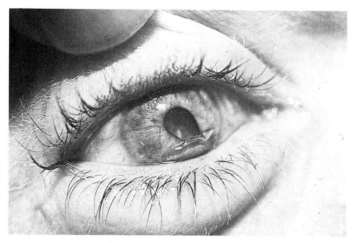

**Fig. 14.5** Perforating corneal wound.

### Patient's needs

- Immediate attention.
- Relief of anxiety about possible loss of the eye.
- Admission to hospital.

### Nursing priorities

- Inform medical staff of the patient's injuries.

### Nursing action

- Allay anxiety.
- Record visual acuity if possible.
- Assist the doctor to examine the eye.
- Clean any wounds around the eye.
- Admit the patient to hospital for:
    (a)   rest and recovery from the accident;
    (b)   pre-operative care prior to excision of prolapsed iris, repair of

corneal wound and restoration of anterior chamber. If the prolapsed iris shows no signs of deterioration and has not been prolapsed for long, it may be repositioned under intensive antibiotic cover.

- Post-operative care. Observe the eye for:
  (a) hyphaema;
  (b) depth of anterior chamber.

## Complications

### *Immediate*

- Loss of anterior chamber.
- Disorganisation of ocular contents.
- Endophthalmitis.

### *Long term*

- Corneal scarring.
- Astigmatism due to scarring.
- Glaucoma.
- Recurrent uveitis.
- Phthisis bulbi.

## 14.9   TRAUMA OF THE UVEAL TRACT

### 14.9.1   Hyphaema (see Fig. 14.6)

Following blunt or penetrating injury to the uveal tract, the iris may bleed into the anterior chamber causing a hyphaema. If, by looking through a slit lamp, the blood cells are seen floating in the anterior chamber, prior to settling inferiorally, this is termed a *microscopic hyphaema*.

A *blackball hyphaema* is one which fills the whole of the anterior chamber.

Sometimes the blood clots in the anterior chamber and may be attached to the iris.

### Patient's needs

- Treatment of the hyphaema by:
  (a) rest at home;
  (b) admission to hospital.

### Nursing action

- Inform medical staff of the patient's condition and history of trauma.
- Admit the patient if necessary.

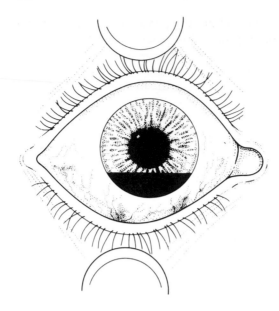

**Fig. 14.6** Hyphaema. (Reproduced with permission from Vaughan, D.G. & Asbury, T. (1983) *General Ophthalmology* (10th edn), Appleton & Lange.)

- Inform the patient of the importance of rest. A severe bleed may occur 48 hours later in a minority of patients, especially if the large ciliary body vessels have bled. The intra-ocular pressure may rise acutely.
- Prepare the patient for an anterior chamber washout in the case of a blackball hyphaema or if the hyphaema has not resolved after 4 to 5 days.
- Give post-operative care. Eye care:
  - (a) instil prescribed drops, e.g. G. chloramphenicol and G. Maxidex (dexamethasone);
  - (b) observe the anterior chamber for depth and recurrence of hyphaema.

    Following a blow to the eye the fundus needs to be examined. There is differing opinion as to whether this should be carried out immediately. Some authorities believe immediate dilation will induce further bleeding (Ragge & Easty 1990).

## Complications

- Secondary bleed 24–48 hours after the initial injury.
- Secondary glaucoma:
  - (a) the blood cells or clot in the anterior chamber blocks the drainage angle;

(b)    angle recession following trauma, which may not become evident for some years, so the patient must have annual eye examinations.

- In long-standing hyphaema the cornea may become blood-stained.

### 14.9.2    Traumatic mydriasis

Following trauma (usually blunt) to the iris, the pupil may become fixed and dilated. This is due to paralysis of the sphincter muscle in the iris. It may resolve itself after a few days. If it is permanent, the patient will experience photophobia.

## 14.10    TRAUMA TO THE LENS

### 14.10.1    Traumatic cataract

Cataract formation can result from a direct or indirect assault on the lens; for example a penetrating injury, such as a hammer and chisel injury, or a blunt injury, such as from a squash ball. An intra-ocular foreign body may lodge on the lens causing a surrounding opacity. This may be the only indication of the intra-ocular foreign body. Trauma to the lens during intra-ocular surgery falls into this category. When the capsule of the lens is injured, aqueous enters the lens substance, causing it to swell and become cloudy. Opacities are most often found in the posterior cortex and sometimes appear like a flower with several petals. They gradually enlarge to cover the whole lens. Lens matter may leak out of the injured capsule into the anterior chamber, where it may cause uveitis or a secondary (phakolytic) glaucoma by blocking the drainage angle. Leaked lens matter can be absorbed by the aqueous, in which case it will not cause any complications.

The development of a traumatic cataract can occur from within a few hours after the incident to months later.

Treatment of a traumatic cataract is similar to that of other causes (see Section 11.2.11).

## 14.11    TRAUMA TO THE RETINA VITREOUS CHOROID AND OPTIC NERVE

Trauma to the posterior segment of the eye may result in a vitreous haemorrhage, retinal tear, retinal detachment (Section 12.6.1), choroidal haemorrhage, choroidal tear, macular tear, optic nerve contusion, or commotio retinae (oedema of the retina).

### 14.11.1  Patient's needs

- Accurate diagnosis and prognosis.
- Preparation for repair of damaged structures (see 'Vitrectomy' and 'Types of retinal detachment surgery' in Section 12.6.1).
- Post-operative care and discharge planning.

### 14.11.2  Nursing action

- Take an accurate history.
- Report to medical staff.
- Assist in examination.
- Allay the patient's anxiety.
- Prepare the patient for surgery as appropriate (see Section 12.6.1).
- Give post-operative care (see Section 12.6.1).
- Plan discharge.

Commotio retinae is managed by rest.

## 14.12  PREVENTION OF OCULAR TRAUMA AND EYE PROTECTION

Nurses working in the ophthalmic casualty area are ideally suited to advise patients on how to prevent ocular trauma. Posters can be displayed in the waiting area and public places outside the hospital that highlight the danger to eyes from certain activities and what protection is available. Eye protection should be worn for racquet sports and for some contact sports as well as in industry. The incidence of ocular trauma has risen with the increase in DIY activities. Suppliers of DIY equipment do not always emphasise the need for eye protection although hire firms are obliged to. There are many types of eye protectors on the market, although some scratch easily or become steamed up. The most effective protectors are more expensive to purchase.

# 15 Removal of an Eye

## 15.1 REMOVAL OF AN EYE

An eye is removed if it is blind and painful, usually as a result of chronic or secondary glaucoma, if there is severe infection or malignancy, or following severe trauma.

There are three operative procedures for removal of an eye.

(1) *Enucleation.* This is the removal of the eyeball itself. It is performed when the eye is blind and painful, following trauma, or for malignancy which is confined to the globe, such as a malignant melanoma of the choroid or retinoblastoma. In cases of malignancy a length of optic nerve must be removed as well to ensure that the disease has not spread along the nerve fibres. If the nerve is found to be involved, radiotherapy will be given to the socket.

(2) *Evisceration* is the removal of the contents of the globe leaving the sclera intact. This is performed following trauma and in cases of severe infection, the sclera being left *in situ* to prevent infection spreading into the brain via the optic nerve and ophthalmic blood vessels.

(3) *Exenteration* is the removal of the total contents of the orbit plus any involved bone. This is performed for malignancy which is outside the eyeball, such as a basal cell carcinoma of the eyelid which has eroded structures behind it.

Removal of the eye should never be performed before a second opinion is obtained as to its necessity.

### 15.1.1 Patient's needs (see Patient Information Leaflet No. 6)

Some patients will already be in hospital following trauma or infection when the decision to remove the eye is taken. Others will need to be admitted. If the eye is blind and painful, the patient may be relieved at the thought of its removal. Some people, though, resist having the eye removed despite severe pain, preferring to rely on analgesics or nerve

---

**PATIENT INFORMATION LEAFLET No. 6**

---

# REMOVAL OF AN EYE

This leaflet is designed to answer some of the questions you may have about having your eye removed, and to emphasise the fact that people are not left with a hole where the eye has been.

### Why do you need to have your eye removed?

There are several reasons why it becomes necessary to remove the eye and it is important that you understand the reason in your case.

The most common reason is that the eye has become painful and blind. The reason for the removal of the eye will be carefully discussed with you by your eye consultant, please feel free to ask as many questions as you wish. If you still have queries when you leave the hospital's outpatients department, please phone your eye consultant's secretary to arrange a further discussion.

### How long will you be in hospital?

This varies but TWO to THREE nights is usual. However if you feel you need to stay longer you can remain in hospital until you feel you can manage at home.

### What kind of anaesthetic will you have?

This depends on your preference and your general health. Most people have a general anaesthetic, which involves being put to sleep for the duration of the operation. Your eye surgeon and the anaesthetist will discuss the options with you.

### When will you have an artificial eye fitted?

Before you leave the hospital you will have a 'shell' fitted into the socket so that its normal shape is retained. You will be taught how to remove, clean and re-insert the shell, if you feel ready to learn. After six weeks you will see the prosthetist who will order you a plastic artificial eye which will be colour matched to your other eye. The plastic eye will be a comfortable fit because a mould will be taken of your socket and the new plastic eye will be shaped to this mould to ensure that it will not cause you any discomfort once fitted. Your 'new eye' will take approximately six weeks to make and you will be fitted with a temporary model meanwhile. The artificial eye will look much like your other eye and will move when the other eye moves. It is often difficult for other people to tell that it is an artificial eye.

### How will your vision be affected?

Looking with one rather than two eyes, reduces your field of view by about one third. You will find it difficult to judge speed of traffic initially, but most people gradually adapt to this.

▶

### PATIENT INFORMATION LEAFLET No. 6 *continued*

#### After your operation

You can go back to your normal life, although you should pay attention to the following points:

#### Drops

You will be given drops or ointments to put in your eye socket for a few weeks after the operation. Detailed instructions will be given to you.

- Always wash your hands before and after instilling the drops and applying the ointment to prevent infection.
- Always shake each bottle before instilling the drops.
- Don't let the bottle tip touch the eye socket.
- Keep on using the drops or ointment until the eye doctor tells you to stop.
- Please bring all drops and ointments to the clinic when you attend.

#### Outpatients appointment

You will normally be seen two weeks after your operation, and once or twice thereafter. If all is well you will then be discharged, and the prosthetist will take over your care.

#### Pain or problems after your operation

If the eye socket aches or becomes sticky in the first two weeks following your discharge, telephone the ward for advice............
Thereafter, telephone Casualty for advice............

#### Work, housework, cooking and gardening

Avoid heavy lifting and straining for two weeks. Otherwise carry on as normal. Most people can return to work two weeks after the operation.

#### Driving

It is best to avoid driving for at least one month after your operation and you should notify the DVLA at Swansea that you have had an eye removed.

#### Bathing

For the first two weeks avoid getting the eye socket wet. You may wash your hair or go to the hairdresser but be careful to avoid getting water in the eye socket.

#### Glasses

It is important that glasses give you the best possible vision in your remaining eye. Please go to your own optician annually for a check-up.

Address:
Anytown Eye Unit
Anytown General Hospital
Any Road
Anytown
AN00 0AN

▶

**PATIENT INFORMATION LEAFLET No. 6** *continued*

**Useful telephone numbers**

Ward . . . . . . . . . . . .
Casualty . . . . . . . . . . . .
Outpatients . . . . . . . . . . .
Orthoptics . . . . . . . . . . . .

blocks for pain relief. It may be worth pointing out to these patients that a blind eye gradually shrinks (phthisis bulbi) and becomes unsightly.

Removal of an eye is an emotive subject and most patients will be highly anxious about the social, physical and psychological effects and will need much support.

The patient's reaction to having an eye removed will vary according to his individual personality, family support, the circumstances surrounding the cause of the removal, his age and sex.

A very young child will not understand fully what is happening and may quickly adapt to a prosthesis as he will have known little else. However, the parents will be feeling very differently, requiring a great amount of support. They may be suffering acute guilt feelings, especially if the child had an accident for which they blame themselves. Siblings and friends may also be upset, especially if they have been involved in, or caused, the accident.

All patients of any age will go through a period of loss for their eye, including feelings of anger and resentment, while coming to terms with their condition. Teenagers may be particularly concerned about their appearance and body image, which may prevent them from socialising with their peers. All age groups and both sexes will be very aware of their changed appearance. They will be much more critical of their prosthesis, noting minute differences to their other eye. It is worth pointing out to them that no two natural eyes in the same face are exactly similar.

Some families and friends will be able to give the patient the necessary support, but others may not feel able to. Some family members may require help from the nurse to come to terms with the patient's loss.

### 15.1.2   Nursing action

- Admit the patient to hospital.
- Give psychological and practical help. Explain about prostheses (see below), pointing out that these days they are very good matches and need not be removed. It may be helpful to put him in touch with a patient who already has a prosthesis. A visit to the prosthetist may benefit the patient.

If the patient is a child, the parents must be totally involved in his care.

- Give pre-operative care.
- Give post-operative care.
  (a) Remove pressure dressing at the first dressing, clean socket and instil prescribed antibiotic ointment. Subsequently the socket will be cleaned regularly and the ointment instilled. No further dressing is applied.
  (b) If the socket is clean, fit a temporary shell into it.
  (c) Teach the patient or parents to remove, clean and replace the shell (see Section 3.2.16), and instil antibiotic ointment.
- On discharge, ensure that the patient has an appointment with the prosthetist and give him the assurance that he can return at any time to the hospital if there are any problems with the shell.

### 15.1.3 Complications

- The socket may become infected at any stage following removal of the eye. This requires cleaning of the socket and antibiotic treatment, usually ointment.
- The socket may shrink with time, causing the prosthesis to protrude, making it appear much larger than the other eye. A new prosthesis will need to be made.

## 15.2 PROSTHESES

Once the initial socket dressing has been removed following surgery and the socket is clean, a temporary shell is inserted into the socket to maintain the shape of the eyelids, to prevent them retracting. The patient is taught to remove, clean and replace this and make sure the socket is clean.

At 4–6 weeks following surgery the patient is fitted with an artificial eye by the prosthetist. This may be fitted earlier if the patient's needs warrant it. Initially a temporary prosthesis is fitted which will match as nearly as possible the patient's other eye. Meanwhile a permanent individualised prosthesis will be made from an impression of the socket. The colour of the sclera, the pattern of the conjunctival vessels, the colour and pattern of the iris and the position of the pupil will be painted on by hand, carefully matching the other eye. Prosthetists are perfectionists in paying attention to the minutest detail.

Prostheses are nowadays made of an inert plastic material which can remain in the socket for up to a year. If there are no problems, the prosthesis is cleaned and polished annually to smooth any rough surfaces.

A prosthesis will need to be removed if it becomes too big for the shrinking socket or if the colour of the other eye changes, as it does with age; the sclera becoming less white and the conjunctival blood vessels more pronounced. The iris may change colour and an arcus senilis may appear.

Prostheses are made to measure and with careful matching of the other eye it is often difficult to tell an artificial eye from a real one (Fig. 15.1). Sometimes the movement of the prosthesis is not as good as in a normal eye. Following an evisceration, movement should be nearly normal as the extra-ocular muscles are still in place and can move the prosthesis. During an enucleation the extra-ocular muscles are cut from their insertion in the sclera and sutured together in the socket. This affords some movement of the prosthesis. Primary socket implantation can be carried out, whereby an acrylic or coralline hydroxyapatite implant is placed in the socket to which the extra-ocular muscles are attached by sutures. This affords more movement of the prosthesis. Implants can be rejected and they tend to extrude after about 20 years, requiring replacement although the hydroxyapatite type aims to overcome this. Being a naturally-derived material from coral, with a similar structure to bone, it is not rejected by the body. The body tissue actually grows into the implant. A peg can be used to attach the prosthesis to the hydroxyapatite implant to afford greater movement of the prosthesis when it is *in situ* (Dutton 1991). After an exenteration, it is not possible to fit a prosthesis into the socket without further plastic surgery. A prosthesis can be attached to spectacles for patients not wishing to undergo further surgery.

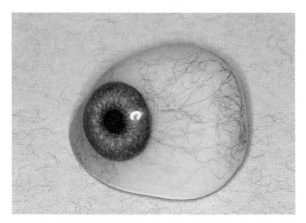

**Fig. 15.1** A prosthesis.

# 16 Ocular Manifestations of Systemic Disease

This chapter summarises the effects of systemic eye disease on the eye. Most of the detailed information has already been discussed and can be found in the chapters on the diseases of the specific ocular structures.

## 16.1 DIABETES MELLITUS (see Patient Information Leaflet No. 7)

Diabetes mellitus can cause the following ocular conditions:

- lids:
  - (a) styes (see Section 5.4.4);
  - (b) chalazions (see Section 5.4.1);
- cornea: keratitis (see Section 8.5);
- iris:
  - (a) rubeosis iridis from neovascularisation (see Section 10.7.3);
  - (b) atrophy of the iris;
  - (c) spontaneous hyphaema from rubeosis iridis;
- chronic open-angle glaucoma;
- secondary glaucoma from rubeosis iridis and peripheral anterior synaechiae (see Section 10.7.3);
- lens:
  - (a) cataract (see Section 11.2.10);
  - (b) intermittent refractive errors due to changes in blood glucose levels and therefore changes in the glucose levels in the lens;
- uveal tract: uveitis (see Section 9.5.2);
- retina:
  - (a) retinal vein occlusion (see Section 12.6.3);
  - (b) retinopathy (see Section 12.6.5);
  - (c) retinal detachment (see Section 12.6.1);
- vitreous: haemorrhage (see Section 12.9.3);
- optic nerve:
  - (a) retrobulbar neuritis (see Section 12.8.2);
  - (b) optic atrophy (see Section 12.8.3);
- nerve palsies. This occurs, rarely, due to inflammation of the third, fourth and sixth cranial nerves causing paralysis of the extra-ocular muscles.

PATIENT INFORMATION LEAFLET No. 7

# DIABETES AND YOUR EYES

### How can diabetes affect your eyes?

Diabetes mellitus can affect your eyes in a number of ways:

- *Diabetic retinopathy*. This occurs in about 30% of all diabetics and can affect your eyesight. It tends to develop after you have had diabetes for a number of years.

- *Cataracts*. Diabetics have an increased risk of developing cataracts but these are unusual in people under 50 years of age.

- *Blurring*. Some diabetics experience temporary blurring of their vision. This is especially likely when their diabetes is poorly controlled and is due to a temporary swelling of the lens in the eye. This may also occur when the diabetes is first treated.

- *Glaucoma*. Diabetics have a slightly increased tendency to develop chronic glaucoma, again this is usually in people aged 60 and above.

### What is diabetic retinopathy?

Diabetes is a disease which principally affects small blood vessels and the body tissues supplied by these blood vessels. Diabetes tends to make these small blood vessels leak so that fats (exudates), fluid (oedema) and blood (haemorrhages) can collect in the retina. The retina lines the inside of the back half of the eye and is responsible for forming an image from the light entering the eye (like a film in a camera). Leaking blood vessels in diabetes can affect your vision (diabetic maculopathy) and may make reading and recognising faces difficult. In addition, blood vessels can become blocked so that the retina does not have an adequate blood supply. As a result, new blood vessels may grow on the surface of the retina. These new vessels are abnormal, tend to bleed and can cause serious eye problems.

### What can you do to help prevent diabetes affecting your eyes?

(1)  Good control of your blood sugar. There is firm evidence to suggest that good control of your diabetes helps prevent diabetic retinopathy.

(2)  No smoking. Smoking considerably increases the risks associated with diabetes. Smokers should therefore seek advice about stopping smoking.

(3)  Control of high blood pressure. If your blood pressure is high consult your family doctor or specialist to ensure that it is well controlled.

(4)  Don't become overweight. Obesity makes diabetes more difficult to control and makes you more likely to develop high blood pressure.

▶

**PATIENT INFORMATION LEAFLET No. 7** *continued*

(5)  Careful monitoring during pregnancy. Diabetic retinopathy can become much worse during pregnancy and requires careful monitoring by an ophthalmologist.

(6)  Have your eyes checked regularly. All diabetics should have their eyes examined once a year. In most cases your hospital specialist or your family doctor should be able to do this. However, if you have developed substantial diabetic changes in your eyes you may need to be seen more frequently and you will probably be under the care of an ophthalmologist.

**What treatment is available for diabetic retinopathy?**

Laser therapy has been shown to be effective in the treatment of diabetic retinopathy. Laser treatment consists of a high energy beam of light which is focused precisely at those areas of the retina which are affected, and so helps prevent the development of sight threatening complications. Laser treatment is given as an outpatient procedure using local anaesthetic drops and a contact lens. The pupils need to be dilated and treatment takes half an hour or less and is usually painless. Most patients have a temporary blurring of vision following laser treatment and it is wise to have someone with you when you go for treatment. Surgery is now possible for very advanced cases of diabetic eye disease but very few people need it.

**For more information**

British Diabetic Association
10 Queen Anne Street
London W1M 0B1
Telephone: 0171 323 1531.

If you have any queries about your diabetes ask one of the doctors or nurses.

Address:
Anytown Eye Unit
Anytown General Hospital
Any Road
Anytown
AN00 0AN

**Useful telephone numbers**

Ward . . . . . . . . . . . .
Casualty . . . . . . . . . . . .
Outpatients . . . . . . . . . . . .
Orthoptics . . . . . . . . . . . .

## 16.2  ACQUIRED IMMUNE DEFICIENCY SYNDROME (AIDS)

AIDS can cause the following conditions:

- microvascular disease:
  - (a)  retina – usually asymptomatic:
    - (i)    cotton wool spots;
    - (ii)   haemorrhages;
    - (iii)  microaneurysms.
  - (b)  conjunctiva – vessels have altered appearance.

- opportunistic infections affecting the retina:
  - (a)  cytomegalovirus (CMV) (see Section 12.6.8);
  - (b)  herpes simplex and zoster;
  - (c)  toxoplasmosis;
  - (d)  Candida;
  - (e)  tuberculosis;
  - (f)  syphilis;
  - (g)  molluscum contagiosum;
  - (h)  Pneumocystis.

- neoplasms:
  - (a)  Kaposi' s sarcoma:
    - (i)    eyelid;
    - (ii)   conjunctiva;
    - (iii)  nose;
    - (iv)  orbit.
  - (b)  Burkitt's lymphoma: orbit.

- neuro-ophthalmic:
  - (a)  cranial nerve palsies;
  - (b)  visual field defects;
  - (c)  papilloedema;
  - (d)  optic atrophy.

## 16.3  THYROID DISEASE

Thyrotoxicosis affects the eye in the following ways (see Section 5.3.4):

- lid lag;
- lid retraction;
- exophthalmos;

- conjunctival chemosis;
- exposure keratitis;
- ophthalmoplegia.

### 16.3.1 Complications

- Corneal ulceration leading to perforation.
- Optic nerve compression.
- Glaucoma.
- Central retinal artery and vein occlusion.
- Cataract.

## 16.4 HYPERTENSION

Hypertension causes a retinopathy (see Section 12.6.5).

## 16.5 GIANT CELL ARTERITIS

Giant cell arteritis or temporal arteritis is a condition of those from the over 60s age group, affecting all arteries, having an effect especially on the heart and kidneys. It is also associated with polymyalgia rheumatica. In the eye it causes a sudden loss of vision in one or both eyes. This is caused by infarctions in the ciliary arteries which supply the optic nerve head causing ischaemia and swelling of the optic disc. The temporal artery is often prominent, hard and tender to touch.

### 16.5.1 Patient's needs

- Relief of symptoms:
  - (a) sudden loss of vision;
  - (b) general malaise;
  - (c) temporal headaches;
  - (d) pain on chewing;
  - (e) tenderness on scalp when combing hair.
- Institution of treatment.

### 16.5.2 Nursing priority

- Inform the doctor of the patient's history of sudden loss of vision.

### 16.5.3 Nursing action

- Instil prescribed mydriatic drops to facilitate ophthalmoscopy.

- Assist the doctor to take blood for ESR estimation. A high reading is indicative of giant cell arteritis. It can be as high as 100 mmHg in one hour.
- Prepare patient and equipment and assist the doctor in performing a temporal artery biopsy. This is not always performed as a false negative result can occur.
- Admit the patient to hospital if the condition is severe enough to warrant high-dose systemic steroids, maybe via the intravenous route.
- If the patient is not admitted, explain the treatment by oral steroids and the importance of carrying a steroid card.
- Ensure the patient has an outpatient follow-up appointment.

High doses of oral steroids are given to prevent further visual loss in the presenting eye if unilateral and to prevent the disease affecting the other eye. These steroids will be gradually reduced and the disease monitored by regular ESR estimations. A maintenance dose of steroids may need to be continued for several years. Patients with severe visual loss resulting from this disease may need to be registered as blind or partially sighted (see Section 1.2).

## 16.6   HERPES SIMPLEX VIRUS (see Section 8.5.3)

Herpes simplex virus causes a conjunctivitis and keratitis resulting in a dendritic corneal ulcer.

## 16.7   HERPES ZOSTER VIRUS (see Section 8.5.3)

In the eye the herpes zoster virus affects the trigeminal nerve. Usually only the ophthalmic branch is involved, but the maxillary branch may be affected too. It causes:

- vesicular eruptions on the forehead, eyelids and nose of affected side of the face, which crust over;
- keratitis;
- conjunctivitis.

### 16.7.1   Complications

- Uveitis.
- Cataract.
- Glaucoma.
- Ophthalmoplegia.
- Persistent pain.

- Ptosis.
- Corneal scarring.
- Anaesthetic cornea.

## 16.8  TUBERCULOSIS

Tuberculosis can cause a uveitis (see Section 9.5.2). Rarely miliary tuberculosis causes discrete yellow nodules in the choroid. A retinitis may develop. Phlyctenular conjunctivitis can be caused by tuberculosis.

## 16.9  SARCOID

Sarcoid can cause a bilateral uveitis (see Section 9.5.2) with mutton fat keratic precipitates present on the corneal endothelium. Dry eyes result from sarcoid involvement of the lacrimal gland (see Section 6.5.4).

## 16.10  SYPHILIS

- Congenital syphilis can cause interstitial keratitis (see Section 8.5.4). It may, rarely, cause a dacryoadenitis.
- Acquired syphilis can cause a uveitis and chorioretinitis.

## 16.11  TOXOPLASMOSIS

The toxoplasma parasite can be transmitted *in utero* if the mother has been infected by ingesting infected meat. It also spreads in the excreta of cats. It causes choroiditis and chorioretinitis (see Section 9.5.1).

## 16.12  TOXOCARA

The toxocara parasite is transmitted via the faeces of puppies and kittens and can cause a unilateral uveitis and choroiditis (see Section 9.5.1) affecting children under the age of 10 years. A chronic endophthalmitis can occur, resulting in severe loss of vision. It can be treated with pyrimethamine and steroids.

## 16.13  RHEUMATOID ARTHRITIS

Rheumatoid arthritis can cause:

- episcleritis (see Section 8.6.2);
- scleritis (see Section 8.6.1);

- uveitis (see Section 9.5.2);
- dry eyes (see Section 6.5.4).

## 16.14   STILLS DISEASE

Stills disease or juvenile rheumatoid arthritis can cause uveitis (see Section 9.5.2).

## 16.15   ANKYLOSING SPONDYLITIS

Ankylosing spondylitis is the main known cause of uveitis (see Section 9.5.2) and scleritis (see Section 8.6.1).

## 16.16   ULCERATIVE COLITIS AND CROHN'S DISEASE

Ulcerative colitis and Crohn's disease can cause uveitis, scleritis and episcleritis (see Sections 9.5.2, 8.6.1 and 8.6.2 respectively).

# 17 Ophthalmic Drugs

This chapter gives brief details of drugs commonly used in ophthalmics.

## 17.1 MYDRIATICS

Mydriatic drugs are used to dilate the pupil for the following reasons:

- to examine the retina;
- to maintain dilation of the pupil in uveitis, with corneal ulcers, severe corneal abrasions and after surgery;
- to break down posterior synaechiae which may be present in uveitis;
- to allow a cataract to be extracted;
- to enable retinal surgery to take place;
- to improve vision when a nuclear cataract is present;
- for refraction in children.

There are two groups of mydriatics:

(1) *parasympatholytics*, which cause mydriasis and cycloplegia – paralysis of the ciliary muscles;
(2) *sympathomimetics*, which cause only mydriasis.

### 17.1.1 Parasympatholytics

**G. + Oc. atropine sulphate** 1%
Derived from the belladonna plant.
*Onset:* 30 minutes.
*Duration:* 7–14 days.
*Dosage:* Usually once or twice a day – may be up to 4 times.
*Side effects:*
(a) may cause an allergic reaction;
(b) toxic effects in the elderly.
*Disadvantages:*
(i) not readily reversed by miotics;

(ii)    prolonged duration;
(iii)   may provoke acute glaucoma in eyes with narrow angle.

**G. homatropine** 1–2%
A man-made derivative of atropine.
*Onset:* 30 minutes.
*Duration:* 24–48 hours.
*Dosage:* 2, 3 or 4 times a day.
*Advantages:*
(a)   can be reversed by pilocarpine;
(b)   shorter duration than atropine.

**G. cyclopentolate hydrochloride** 0.5–1% (Mydrilate)
*Onset:* 30 minutes.
*Duration:* 24 hours.
*Dosage:* 2, 3 or 4 times a day.
*Uses:* often used in refraction of children. Pre- and post-operatively.

**G. tropicamide** 0.5–1% (Mydriacyl)
*Onset:* 20 minutes.
*Duration:* 6 hours.
*Dosage:* usually only once before examination because of its short-lived effect.
*Advantage:* short duration makes it suitable for ophthalmoscopy in out-patient or casualty patients.

### 17.1.2   Sympathomimetics

**G. adrenaline**
Although adrenaline is a mydriatic it is rarely used as such. It can be used as a conjunctival decongestant as it is also vasoconstrictive. A weak solution, 0.5%–1%, is used in the treatment of open-angle glaucoma (see Section 17.3).

**G. phenylephrine** 2.5–10%
*Onset:* 20 minutes.
*Duration:* 3 hours.
*Dosage:* 2, 3, or 4 times daily, or up to 4-hourly to break down posterior synaechiae.
*Use:* Effective in combination with parasympatholytics, especially in the breaking down of posterior synaechiae.
*Disadvantages:*
(a)   it does not cause cycloplegia;
(b)   it can cause corneal epithelial damage;
(c)   may cause cardiovascular reactions that may be severe.

### 17.1.3  Notes on mydriatics

(1)  Mydriatics must be used with care in patients who have shallow anterior chambers as dilating the pupils may provoke an attack of closed-angle glaucoma.
(2)  All mydriatics drops sting on instillation to some degree. Phenylephrine usually causes the most discomfort.

## 17.2  MIOTICS

Miotic drugs constrict the pupil and the ciliary muscle which opens up the drainage channel for aqueous flow. Therefore their main use is in the treatment of glaucoma.

**G. pilocarpine** 0.25–6% (may be up to 10% in other parts of the world)
A natural compound from the pilocarpes tree found in South America. It is a parasympathomimetic.
*Onset:* 30 minutes.
*Duration:* 10–12 hours.
*Dosage:* 2 , 3, or 4 times a day, or intensively for acute glaucoma.
*Disadvantages:*
(a)  can cause headaches;
(b)  the eye is fixed at accommodation;
(c)  the pupil remains permanently miosed,
(d)  care must be taken when used intensively as overdose can cause vomiting;
(e)  may cause an allergic reaction;
(f)  can sting on instillation.

**Acetylcholine chloride** 1% (Miochol)
A freshly prepared solution of acetylcholine is injected into the anterior chamber after a cataract extraction to constrict the pupil rapidly to prevent vitreous loss, or to retain a posterior chamber or iris clip intra-ocular lens in position.

## 17.3  OTHER DRUGS USED IN THE TREATMENT OF GLAUCOMA

### 17.3.1  Carbonic anhydrase inhibitors

Carbonic anhydrase is an enzyme necessary for the production of aqueous. These drugs therefore cause a reduction in the amount of aqueous produced.

**Acetazolamide** (Diamox)
*Dosage:*
(a)   500 mg intravenously stat in acute glaucoma;
(b)   500 mg orally stat;
(c)   250 mg orally as maintenance 4 times a day reducing to 3 or 2 doses a
       day or slow release capsules 250 mg given once or twice a day.
*Uses:* in acute, chronic and secondary glaucoma.
*Side effects:* drowsiness, gastro-intestinal upset, nausea and potassium loss
resulting in tingling of extremities. Potassium supplements such as
potassium chloride are sometimes given. It is a weak diuretic.

**Dichlorphenamide** 50 mg (Daranide)
*Dosage:* initially 100–200 mg. Then 100 mg twice a day.
*Maintenance dose:* 25–50 mg, 1, 2 or 3 times a day.
It is often used if patients are intolerant to acetazolamide.

**Dorzolamide** 2% (Trusopt)
*Dosage:* 3 times a day, or twice a day if given with a beta-blocker.
*Use:* in chronic and secondary glaucoma as an adjuvant therapy to beta-
blockers or as a single therapy to non-responders or in those who are
unable to tolerate beta-blockers.
*Side effects:* conjunctivitis, eyelid irritation.

### 17.3.2   Beta-blockers

**G. timolol maleate** 0.25–0.5% (Timoptol)
**G. betaxolol hydrochloride** 0.5% (Betoptic)
**G. carteolol hydrochloride** 1% (Teoptic)
**G. levobunolol hydrochloride** 0.5% (Betagan).
*Actions:* reduce the production of aqueous and after several weeks' use
increase the outflow of aqueous.
*Dosage:* 12 hourly, strictly. (Betagan may be used daily.)
*Advantages:* do not cause miosis or accommodation spasm.
*Disadvantages:* cannot be used in patients with a history of asthma or
congestive cardiac failure.
Timolol and levobunolol are available in single dose presentations.

### 17.3.3   Other drugs

**G. adrenaline** 1% (Eppy) or 0.5%, 1% (Simplene)
*Action:* Reduces aqueous formation and after several weeks' use increases
the outflow of aqueous.

*Dosage:* twice a day.
*Use:* for open-angle glaucoma.
*Disadvantages:*
(a)  burning on administration;
(b)  slight mydriatic effect which might blur the vision;
(c)  pigmented spots develop in the conjunctiva.

**G. dipivefrine** 0.1% (Propine)
*Action:* reduces aqueous formation and after several weeks' use increases aqueous outflow.
*Dosage:* twice a day.
*Advantages:* a prodrug which penetrates the cornea more readily than adrenaline and breaks down to adrenaline in the eye.

**Mannitol** 20%
*Use:* given intravenously in acute glaucoma when acetazolamide has failed to reduce the intra-ocular pressure. It can be given pre-operatively. Usually 1.5–2 g/kg body weight is given over 1 hour.

**Glycerol**
*Action:* an osmotic.
*Use:* oral dose given in acute glaucoma when acetazolamide has failed to reduce the intra-ocular pressure.
*Dosage:* 1.5 g/kg body weight in fruit juice to disguise the taste. It must be drunk within 20 minutes to affect the intra-ocular pressure. Topical glycerol 50% can be used to clear corneal oedema temporarily for ophthalmoscopy to take place.

**G. apraclonidine hydrochloride** 0.5% and 1% (Iopidine)
*Action:* reduces production of aqueous.
*Use:* adjunctive therapy in chronic glaucoma.
*Dosage:* 3 times a day.
*Side effects:* it is contraindicated in patients with severe or unstable cardiovascular disease, those receiving monoamine oxidase inhibitors, sympathomimetic drugs and tricyclic antidepressants. Localised allergy.


## 17.4  ANTIBIOTICS

**Chloramphenicol guttae** 0.5%, Oc. 1%.
*Action:* bacteriostatic, broad spectrum.
*Uses:* in ocular infections. It can penetrate the corneal epithelium. Prophylactic use.
*Dosage:* 2-hourly or 2, 3, or 4 times a day.
*Advantage:* resistance is slow to develop.

**Gentamicin** 0.3% (Genticin) (drops and ointment) 1.5% fortified.
*Action:* bactericidal, broad spectrum.
*Uses:* ocular infections resistant to chloramphenicol. For *Pseudomonas aeruginosa* infections.
*Dosage:* 2-hourly or 2, 3, or 4 times a day.
*Subconjunctival injection:* 20 mg.

**Neomycin sulphate** 0.5% (drops and ointment)
*Action:* bactericidal, broad spectrum.
*Uses:* in conjunctivitis, blepharitis, superficial infections.
*Dosage:* 2-hourly or 2 or 4 times a day.
*Disadvantages:*
(a)   it does not penetrate corneal tissue;
(b)   it may cause an allergic reaction.

**Framycetin sulphate** 0.5% drops or ointment (Soframycin)
Action, uses and dosage similar to neomycin and therefore can be given in cases allergic to neomycin.

**G. penicillin** 0.3%
*Action:* broad spectrum, antibiotic.
*Dosage:* intensively for severe infection, or 2, 3, or 4 times a day.
*Uses:* in corneal ulcers, ophthalmia neonatorum, hypopyon ulcer.
*Disadvantages:*
(a)   unstable and cannot be stored for long periods;
(b)   may cause an allergic reaction;
(c)   not commercially available.

**Chlortetracycline** (Aureomycin) 1%
*Action:* bacteriostatic, broad spectrum.
*Dosage:* 4 times a day.
*Uses:* in conjunctivitis, especially trachoma, blepharitis, ophthalmia neonatorum, dacryocystitis.
*Disadvantage:* does not penetrate corneal epithelium.

**G. ciprofloxacin** 0.3%
*Action:* broad spectrum antibiotic.
*Dosage:* intensively for severe infections or 2, 3, or 4 times a day.
*Uses:* corneal ulcers, especially caused by pseudomonas.
*Side effects:* local burning and itching, lid margin crusting.

**Fucidic acid** 1% (Fucithalmic)
*Action:* broad spectrum antibiotic.
*Dosage:* usually twice a day.
*Uses:* superficial infections.

*Advantages:* a viscid substance that is not absorbed as readily as drops and therefore need not be administered as frequently. Useful in children.

**G. cefuroxine** 5%
*Action:* broad spectrum antibiotic.
*Dosage:* intensively for severe infection or 2, 3, or 4 times a day.
*Uses:* corneal ulcers, ophthalmic neonatorum, hypopyon ulcer.
*Disadvantages:*
(a)   not very stable;
(b)   needs refrigeration;
(c)   not commercially available.

## 17.5   ANTIVIRAL AGENTS

**Oc. aciclovir** (Zovirax) 3%
*Dosage:* 5 times a day.
*Uses:* in herpes simplex virus and herpes zoster ophthalmicus. A cream preparation 5% is available for use on skin lesions.

**G. trifluorthymidine** 1% (F3T)
*Dosage:* 5 times a day.
*Uses:* as an alternative to Aciclovir for herpes simplex ulcers and stromal keratitis.
*Disadvantages:*
(a)   not commercially available;
(b)   must be kept refrigerated.

**G. propamidine isethionate** 0.1% (Brolene)
*Use:* in acanthamoeba keratitis.
*Dosage:* 4 times a day.
*Disadvantage:* little value in bacterial conjunctivitis.

## 17.6   STEROIDS

Steroid drops are used for:

* allergic conditions;
* with an antibiotic in bacterial inflammatory conditions, e.g. chronic conjunctivitis;
* inflammatory conditions such as uveitis, sympathetic ophthalmia, episcleritis.

**G. prednisolone** (Predsol) 0.001%–0.5% (1% Prod. Forte)
*Dosage:* 4 times a day.

**Methylprednisolone** (Depo-Medrone) 20 mg
*Dosage:* 1 dose subconjunctivally.
Must not be mixed with other drugs in the same syringe. Will leave a white deposit under the conjunctiva for up to 3 weeks.

**Betamethasone** (Betnesol) G. and Oc. 0.1%
*Dosage:* 2 hourly, 2, 3, or 4 times a day, ointment at night. 2–4 mg sub-conjunctivally.

**G. hydrocortisone** 1% (ointment 0.5%, 1%, 2.5%)
*Dosage:* 4 times a day, ointment at night.

**G. dexamethasone** (Maxidex) 0.1%
*Dosage:* hourly – 2-hourly if needed intensively, frequency gradually reducing, or 2 or 4 times a day. Must be shaken before instillation.

**G. clobetasone** 0.1% (Eumovate)
*Dosage:* 2 or 4 times a day with reducing frequency.
Used as alternative steroid preparation as it is said not to raise the intraocular pressure as much as other topical steroids (see below).

**Neomycin** can be combined with a steroid.
**Predsol-N** (prenisolone 0.5% and neomycin 0.5%).
**Betnesol-N** (betamethasone 0.1% and neomycin 0.5%) drops and ointment.
**Maxitrol** (dexamethasone 0.1%, neomycin 0.5% and Polymyxin B)
**Eumovate-N** (clobetasone 0.1% and neomycin 0.5%).
**Chloramphenicol** 1% and **hydrocortisone** 1% in ointment preparation.

### 17.6.1   Disadvantages of steroid use

* Lowers the resistance to microorganisms.
* Masks signs of infection.
* Increases the activity of herpes simplex virus.
* May cause herpes simplex viral infection if prescribed for conjunctivitis.
* May cause secondary glaucoma.
* Prolonged use may cause cataract formation.

## 17.7   LOCAL ANAESTHETICS

**G. cocaine** 4%
*Dosage:* 1 drop at 5 minute intervals over 20–25 minutes.
*Use:* prior to surgery under local anaesthesia.

*Disadvantages:*
(a)  it may cause clouding of the corneal epithelium;
(b)  the pupil may become dilated;
(c)  it may cause a systemic reaction (weak rapid pulse, confusion, vomiting).

### G. amethocaine 4%
*Dosage:* 1 drop at 2–3 minute intervals over 20 minutes.
*Use:* prior to surgery under local anaesthesia.
*Disadvantage:* causes stinging on initial instillation.

### Oxybruprocaine hydrochloride 0.4% (Benoxinate)
*Dosage:* usually once only is sufficient.
*Use:* prior to minor ophthalmic procedures.

### G. proxymetacaine 0.5% (Ophthaine)
*Dosage:* usually once only is sufficient.
*Use:* minor ophthalmic procedures, often used in children due to reduced stinging on instillation.

## 17.8   DIAGNOSTIC DROPS

### Fluorescein
*Drops* 2%.
*Uses:*
(a)  stains conjunctival and corneal epithelial damage, i.e. corneal ulcers, erosions and conjunctival or corneal abrasions;
(b)  assessment of the tear film;
(c)  tonometry;
(d)  Seidel's test shows fluorescein-stained aqueous leaking from a wound on the cornea/limbus;
(e)  contact lens fitting.
Fluorescein is also available in paper strips.
   Fluorescein should not be dispensed in a multiple container as it is a good medium for *Pseudomonas* bacterial growth.

*Intravenous* 20%
*Use:* for fundal fluorescein angiography, which demonstrates the condition of the retinal blood vessels, the condition of the macula and optic disc and the presence of choroidal tumours.

### G. rose bengal 1%
*Use:* stains dead conjunctival and corneal epithelium in dry eye syndrome.

*Disadvantage:* painful on instillation and the eye should be irrigated following its use.


## 17.9   TEAR REPLACEMENT

The following are used for dry eyes and must be used as often as is necessary to keep the eyes feeling comfortable. This may be as often as every hour. Once dry eyes have been diagnosed the patient may need to continue to use tear replacement drops for life.
**G. hypromellose.**
**G. Tears Naturale.**
**G. Liquifilm Tears.**
**G. Viscotears** (long-acting gel formulation)
**Simple eye ointment**
**oc. Lacri-Lube.**


## 17.10   MISCELLANEOUS

**G. antazoline sulphate 0.5%**
**Xylometazoline hydrocloride** 0.05% (G. Otrivine Antistin)
*Use:* in allergic conjunctivitis, especially caused by hay fever, for short-term use only.
*Dosage:* 2 or 3 times a day.


**G. sodium cromoglycate** (Opticrom) 2%
*Use:* in allergic conjunctivitis, especially vernal catarrh.
*Dosage:* 4 times a day.


**G. lodoxamide** (Alomide) 0.1%
*Use:* in allergic conjunctivitis, as an alternative to Opticrom.
*Dosage:* 4 times daily.


**Sodium hyaluronate** (Healonid)
A visco-elastic polymer normally present in aqueous.
*Use:* during surgical procedures to protect internal structures and maintain depth of anterior chamber.
*Side effects:* occasional hypersensitivity, transient rise in intra-ocular pressure.


**Hydroxypropylmethylecellulose** (HPMC)
*Use:* during surgery to protect internal structures and maintain depth of anterior chamber.

**Botulinum toxin** (*clostridium botulinum* type A; Dysport, Botox)
*Action:* paralysis of muscles.
*Use:* to treat blepharospasm and strabismus and to induce ptosis to protect the cornea.
*Dosage:* varies depending on use and which product is used.
*Side effects:* as it is a biological product, anaphylaxis may occur.

**Diclofenac sodium** 0.1% (Volterol Ophtha)
*Use:* inhibits intra-operative miosis, reduces post-cataract surgery inflammation.
*Dosage:*
(a)  pre-operative: $\frac{1}{2}$ hourly four times;
(b)  post-operative: 4 times a day.
*Advantage:* preservative-free preparation.

## 17.11   GENERAL NOTE

Some ophthalmic drugs are prepared in single-dose containers which contain no preservative. Therefore they are useful for those patients who may be allergic to the preservative used in ophthalmic preparations.

# Appendix 1: Correction of Refractive Errors

Light travels in rays which are reflected from objects into the eyes. Light rays travel in straight lines from a distance of 6 metres or more. At a shorter distance they diverge as they enter the eye. When light rays meet a transparent object at an angle they bend. This is called 'refraction'. Light rays entering the eye meet the curved cornea and bend inwards or converge. They continue to converge as they pass through each of the refractive media of the eye, the cornea, the aqueous, the lens and the vitreous, so that they are brought to a focal point on the retina.

The 'refractive power' of the eye is the degree to which the eye is able to refract the light rays. This power is expressed in dioptres. One dioptre brings rays of light to a focus over one metre. Ten dioptres bring rays of light to a focus over one-tenth of a metre or 10 cm. The refractive power of the eye is 60 dioptres, that of the lens is 20 dioptres and of the cornea 40 dioptres.

## A1.1   LONG SIGHT OR HYPERMETROPIA

A long-sighted person has a short eyeball. The light rays therefore come to a focus behind the retina causing blurred vision. A long-sighted person consequently has to accommodate for distant vision to be clear. No further accommodation is possible for near vision, so this is blurred. If a convex lens is placed in front of the eye, the light rays will converge more sharply and come to a focus on the retina. A convex lens is a spherical lens because its shape is equal in all meridians. It is known as a 'plus' lens.

## A1.2   SHORT SIGHT OR MYOPIA

A short-sighted person has a long eyeball. The light rays therefore come to a focus in front of the retina. The vision is usually more blurred for distant vision than near vision as the lens can accommodate for near vision. If a concave lens is placed in front of the eye, the light rays will diverge before converging through the cornea and lens and will come to a focus at the retina. A concave lens is also spherical and is known as a 'minus' lens.

Iris claw lenses have been placed in phakic eyes above –6.00 dioptres myopia with successful results (Menezo *et al.* 1995).

## A1.3   PRESBYOPIA

From the age of about 45 years, the lens in the eye no longer has the ability to accommodate for near vision. The light rays therefore fall behind the retina before coming to a focus. This is known as presbyopia. Convex or plus lenses are needed to bring the image into focus on the retina. An increasingly powerful lens is required until the age of 70 years when no further deterioration in focusing occurs.

## A1.4   ASTIGMATISM

The astigmatic cornea has an uneven curvature so that there is no point of focus of the light rays on the retina. A cylindrical lens placed in front of the eye with its axis corresponding to the abnormal plane on the cornea will focus the light rays. The cylindrical lens can either be concave or convex.

Most spectacles combine both spherical (plus or minus) lenses with cylindrical lenses to provide a compound lens to correct myopia/ hypermetropia and astigmatism. Full information on optics is beyond the scope of this book.

## A1.5   REFRACTIVE SURGERY

In recent years there has been an increased interest in refractive surgery. Initially this was performed for myopia, but recent advances have enabled patients with hypermetropia and astigmatism also to be treated. It is still at an early stage of development and the long-term results are unknown. There is a degree of controversy and caution about the process (Gartry 1995).

### A1.5.1   Patient's needs

- The patient must have detailed explanations given of the procedure itself and any complications.
- Topography investigations. The curvature of the cornea is measured in detail resulting in a coloured map of the cornea. Areas that are too flat are coloured blue and those too steep red. The ideal curvature is green.
- Pre- and post-operative care.
- Follow-up information.

## A1.5.2    Nursing action

- Assist/perform topography.
- Ensure the patient has a full understanding of the procedure and that he does not have unrealistic expectations.
- Give pre-operative care. Local anaesthetic drops will be instilled.
- Assist in the laser surgery.
- Give post-operative care:
    (a)   a bandage contact lens will be in place (see Section A2.2.3);
    (b)   ensure the patient has adequate analgesia;
    (c)   ensure the patient has follow-up information including understanding that if treated for myopia, he will initially be hypermetropic.

## A1.5.3    Types of surgery

The surgery uses laser and is constantly changing as technology improves.

### Excimer laser photorefractive keratectomy (PRK)

A computer estimates the depth and position of the corneal tissue to be removed which will vary depending on the refractive error being treated. The epithelium is removed before the laser ablates the cornea.
    Shortcomings of the procedure are:

- visual results are better predicted in patients whose refractive error is less than – 6 dioptres than higher myopes (– 6 to – 10). However, higher myopes can obtain a reduction in their myopia (Carson & Taylor 1995);
- severe pain while the epithelium regenerates;
- complications include: corneal haze which is significantly more in myopes greater than – 10 (Carson & Taylor 1995), regression, loss of best corrected visual acuity, night halo effects, wound infection, delayed healing and perforation.

### Combined excimer laser and micro surgery

A micro layer of corneal tissue from under the epithelium is shaved off prior to laser application and the epithelium is replaced. This reduces the problems of pain, corneal haze and regression.

## A1.6    PARALYTIC SQUINT

When a paralytic squint occurs, the image to each eye is not focusing on the same area of each retina. If a prism is placed in front of the squinting eye, the light rays bend towards the base of the triangular-shaped prismatic lens and will cause the image to focus in the area of the retina of that eye corresponding to the area of retina in the other eye. This results in a single image being seen or binocular single vision.

# Appendix 2: Contact Lenses

## A2.1 USES OF CONTACT LENSES

- *Refractive errors.* People may wear contact lenses for cosmetic reasons instead of glasses. High myopes benefit from wearing contact lenses because they would need to wear thick-lensed glasses which cause visual distortion. Contact lenses afford much improved vision involving the whole visual field.
- *Aphakia* (see Section 11.3).
- *Corneal abnormalities* such as keratoconus (see Section 8.5.7).
- *Protection.* A bandage lens can protect the eye from perforating or becoming too dry. Painted contact lenses are worn by albinos or people with aniridia to prevent too much light entering the eye.

## A2.2 TYPES OF LENS

- Hard lens.
- Gas-permeable lens.
- Soft lens.
- Extended-wear lens.
- Bandage lens.
- Disposable – weekly/daily.
- Toric for astigmatism.
- Bifocal.

### A2.2.1 Hard and gas-permeable lenses

Hard and gas-permeable lenses must be removed before sleep or if the eye is irritable. If they are kept in under these circumstances, corneal damage is likely to occur. Artificial teardrops may be required to prevent the cornea drying out. Gas-permeable lenses should cause less corneal dryness.

## A2.2.2  Soft lenses

Soft lenses are slightly larger than hard lenses. They tend to be used if the wearer finds hard lenses intolerable. They should also be removed at night and if the eye is irritable. More scrupulous care is required for soft lenses as they are more likely to cause corneal damage; because they are made of a softer material than hard lenses, a scratch on the cornea or a small foreign body underneath the lens is not so likely to be felt until damage has been done.

Fluorescein drops should never be put into an eye with a soft contact lens in, as the dye will be taken up by the lens and is extremely difficult, if not impossible, to remove. Only eyedrops without preservative should be used with soft contact lenses, as the preservative can be absorbed by the lens, which may provoke an allergic reaction. Soft lenses should be stored in normal saline if no soaking solution is available; water, whether sterile or not, will cause them to dry out.

## A2.2.3  Extended-wear lenses and bandage lenses

Extended-wear lenses and bandage lenses are essentially similar to soft lenses but are larger in size. They can be worn for up to 3 months without being removed, so are therefore useful for the young and the elderly. The optician removes the lens and cleans it by a boiling process before reinserting it. Artificial teardrops will be required to prevent the cornea drying out.

Bandage lenses do not have a prescription incorporated.

## A2.2.4  Disposable/weekly lenses

Disposable lenses are becoming more popular. Initially the lenses were designed to be worn day and night for 6 days and then discarded. The eyes were rested on the seventh day. Some contact lens wearers now use disposable lenses but as daily wear, removing them at night to reduce the complications (see Section A2.5).

## A2.3  CARE OF CONTACT LENSES

Contact lenses require great care to prevent corneal damage and eye infection. There are several different brands of products on the market for use with contact lenses. There are different solutions for hard and soft lenses.

Care of lenses involves:

- *cleansing* with a cleansing solution rubbed on the lens with the finger and washed off with water. It has been suggested that using solutions

containing hydrogen peroxide are better in that they destroy acanthamoeba (see Section A2.5);

- *wetting* – wetting solution is dropped onto the corneal surface of the
  lens before it is inserted into the eye;
- *soaking the lens* – when the lens is not in the eye, i.e. overnight, it is
  placed in a special container filled with soaking solution. This fluid
  should be changed each time the container is used. Once a week the
  container should be washed out with warm water and rinsed with the
  soaking solution.

Lenses should be cleaned well and checked by an optician before being
re-inserted following corneal damage.

## A2.4    INSERTION/REMOVAL OF CONTACT LENSES

See Section 3.2.15 for details of how to insert and remove contact lenses.

## A2.5    COMPLICATIONS OF CONTACT LENS WEAR

- *Intolerance.* Some people find wearing contact lenses intolerable. Hard
  lenses are usually prescribed initially as they cause less problems. If
  these are difficult to wear, gas-permeable or soft contact lenses are
  prescribed. Some people have to abandon contact lens wearing and
  resort to spectacles.
- *Dry eyes.* The lens prevents the tear film from adequately covering the
  cornea. Artificial teardrops can be prescribed for people who do
  experience dry eyes.
- *Giant papillary conjunctivitis or contact lens associated papillary conjunctivitis.* This is more common in wearers of soft contact lenses. It
  may not manifest itself for months or years after starting to wear
  lenses.
    Symptoms include:
  (a)    itching;
  (b)    mucus discharge;
  (c)    increasing intolerance to lens wear.
    Sign: large conjunctival papillae (Allansmith *et al.* 1977).
- *Hypoxia.* The cornea is deprived of oxygen from the tear film by the
  presence of the contact lens. The cornea becomes oedematous and new
  vessels may develop in the limbal area. This usually occurs after years
  of contact lens wear.
- *Sensitivity.* This may develop in response to the preservative in the
  cleaning and soaking solutions.
- *Keratitis.* People wearing extended-wear soft contact lenses are 21

times more likely to get microbial keratitis than gas-permeable lens wearers and daily soft contact lens wearers are four times more likely (Cochrane 1993). *Acanthamoeba* is the most dangerous organism requiring intensive antibiotic application (Seal & Hay 1992). This may be neomycin and propamidine. The contact lens should not be reinserted into the eye until the infection has cleared and the lens itself has been cleaned.

It is advisable for all contact lens wearers to have a spare pair of spectacles to wear in case they are unable to use their contact lenses for a while.

## A2.6   NURSE'S ROLE

Although nurses do not prescribe or fit contact lenses, they are in an ideal position to educate people on the care of contact lenses whether the

---

**ADVICE SHEET No. 8**
**Eye Casualty Department**

# CARE OF YOUR CONTACT LENSES

Contact lenses must be worn with care. Always follow the instructions and advice of your optician.

**Main points**

(1) Do not wear 'disposable' lenses at night. They do not allow enough oxygen through the cornea (the front of the surface of the eye) to keep it healthy.

(2) Make sure you visit your optician regularly to have your soft lenses sterilised and checked before reinserting them. If you wear hard contact lenses attend your fitter at the recommended intervals.

(3) Make sure you clean your contact lens case thoroughly and change it regularly as recommended by your optician.

(4) Always have a pair of glasses for use in an emergency.

(5) If your eye is sore take your lens out immediately and seek help.

(6) Having visited the Eye Casualty follow the instructions of the doctor or nurse. If the eye does not improve please ring the department for further advice.

person has a problem or in a more informal advisory capacity (see Advice Sheet No. 8).

Nurses must stress the importance of the following:

- complying with scrupulous and effective care regimes of their contact lenses (Wakelin 1995). However, wearers of extended-wear soft contact lenses have an increased risk of keratitis despite complying with hygiene instructions (Stapleton 1992);
- the need to discard any solutions after 28 days of use;
- saliva and tap water must not be used as wetting or cleaning solutions;
- other people's contact lens cases, which may not be clean, must not be 'borrowed' for their lenses;
- allowing time for the cornea to 'breathe' by removing the lenses for a period of time each day;
- removal of lenses, except extended-wear lenses, at night;
- washing of hands prior to handling lenses and avoiding creamy soft soaps and ensuring all traces of hand cream are removed from finger tips.

# Index of Symptoms

| Symptom | Structure involved |
|---|---|
| *Blur* | |
| If the blur is cleared by wearing glasses, by partly closing the eyes or by blinking. | Cornea – astigmatism<br>Lens – opacity<br>Lacrimal system – deficient tear film<br>Conjunctiva – (a) discharge from conjunctivitis; (b) foreign body or foreign sensation causing watering eye<br>Cornea – foreign body or abrasion causing watering eye |
| If there is a constant fog or haze | Cornea – opacity<br>Lens opacity<br>Vitreous – opacity<br>Macula – maculopathy |
| *Central scotoma* | Macula – degeneration<br>Optic nerve – (a) atrophy; (b) neuritis; (c) retrobulbar neuritis<br>Optic pathways – lesion |
| *Diplopia*<br>With both eyes open | Extra-ocular muscles or their nerve supply – paralytic squint |
| Uni-ocular | Lens – opacity |
| *Discharge* | Lids – blepharitis<br>Conjunctiva – bacterial conjunctivitis<br>Cornea – ulcer<br>Lacrimal drainage system – dacryocystitis |

*Dryness*

Lacrimal gland ⎫
Lids            ⎬  deficient
Conjunctiva    ⎭  tear film

*Epiphora*

Lacrimal drainage system – blocked
    duct
Meibomian gland in lid – lack of oil
    layer of tear film
Foreign body
Conjunctiva – viral conjunctivitis
Lid margin – ectropion

*Floaters*

Vitreous – (a) haemorrhage;
    (b) detachment; (c) syneresis

*Glare*

Cornea – opacity
Lens – opacity
Retina – diabetic retinopathy

*Itching*

Lid – allergy
Conjunctiva – allergic conjunctivitis

*Pain*
Foreign body sensation

Conjunctiva – (a) bacterial and viral
    infection; (b) pinguecula;
    (c) pterygium; (d) foreign body;
    (e) episcleritis
Cornea – (a) foreign body; (b) abrasion;
    (c) ulcer

Deep pain

Ciliary body/iris – uveitis
Optic nerve – (a) neuritis;
    (b) retrobulbar neuritis
Orbit – cellulitis

*Peripheral field defect*
Monocular – patient usually aware of
    the symptoms

Retina – (a) central retinal artery or vein
    occlusion; (b) detachment
Optic nerve – atrophy

Bilateral – patient
often unaware of symptoms

Optic nerve – chronic glaucoma
Optic pathways – lesion

*Photophobia*

Cornea – (a) foreign body; (b) abrasion;
    (c) ulcer
Ciliary body/iris – uveitis
Iris – lack of pigment, e.g. albinism
Retina – retinitis pigmentosa

# Glossary

**Abduction**   Turning the eye outwards.

**Acanthamoeba**   A genus of free-living amoeba.

**Accommodation**   The ability of the lens to change shape to allow near objects to be focused on the retina.

**Adduction**   Turning the eye inwards.

**Amblyopia**   Reduced vision usually due to interference with the eye's development.

**Angles Alpha, Kappa and Gamma**   Different angles in the eye measured between the optic axis and the visual axis.

**Aniridia**   Absence of the iris.

**Aphakia**   Absence of the lens.

**Applanation tonometry**   Measurement of the intra-ocular pressure by flattening the cornea.

**Arcus senilis**   Degenerative change in the cornea resulting in a white ring around the corneal circumference.

**Argon laser**   Laser that uses photocoagulation.

**Astigmatism**   Uneven curvature of the cornea.

**Binocular vision**   Coordinated use of both eyes resulting in a single vision.

**Biometry**   Measurement of the axial length of the eye (A-scan).

**Blepharitis**   Inflammation of the lid margin.

**Blepharospasm**   Painful involuntary spasm of the eyelids.

**Blind spot**   Optic disc where there are no nerve endings, only nerve fibres.

**Bullous keratopathy**   Oedema of the cornea causing 'blister' formation in the epithelium.

**Canthus**   Outer and inner areas where the upper and lower lids meet.

**Capsulotomy**   Opening of the capsule of the lens.

**Cartella shield**   Plastic shield to protect the eye.

**Caruncle**   Small fleshy area in inner corner of the eye.

**Cataract**   Opacity of the lens.

**Central field/vision**   Area of vision when looking straight ahead.

**Chalazion**   Meibomian gland cyst. Internal hordeolum.

**Chemosis**   Oedema of the conjunctiva.

**Chlamydia**   Chronic conjunctivitis caused by serotypes D–K of *Chlamydia trachomatis*.

**Commotio retinae**   Oedema of the retina following trauma.

**Concave lens**   A lens which diverges light rays, used to correct myopia: a 'minus' lens.
**Concretion**   Lipid deposit in the conjunctiva.
**Convex lens**   A lens which converges light rays, used to correct hypermetropia: a 'plus' lens.
**Cycloplegia**   Paralysis of the ciliary muscles.
**Cylindrical lens**   A lens of cylindrical shape, which refracts light rays in various directions in different meridians, used to correct astigmatism.

**Dacryoadenitis**   Inflammation of the lacrimal gland.
**Dacryocystitis**   Inflammation of the lacrimal sac.
**Dacryocystorhinostomy**   An operation to make a passage from the lacrimal sac into the nose to overcome an obstruction.
**Dendritic ulcer**   A branching ulcer of the cornea caused by the herpes simplex virus.
**Descemetocele**   Protrusion of Descemet's membrane through the stroma and epithelium of the cornea.
**Dioptre**   Unit of measurement of strength of the refractive power of the eye, or lenses, expressed as a fraction of a metre.
**Diplopia**   Double vision.
**Disciform keratitis**   Inflammation of the cornea as a complication of herpes simplex virus.
**Distichiasis**   Double row of eyelashes.
**Drusen**   Small yellow nodule in Bruch's membrane, or optic nerve.

**Ectropion**   Turning out of the eyelid.
**Electroretinogram**   A recording of electrical activity of the retina.
**Emmetropia**   Absence of refractive error.
**Endophthalmitis**   Inflammation/infection of inner structures of the eye.
**Enophthalmos**   Displacement of the eyeball downwards.
**Entropion**   Turning inwards of the lid margin.
**Enucleation**   Removal of the eyeball and length of optic nerve.
**Epicanthus**   Broad fold of skin in inner canthus.
**Epilation**   Removal of an eyelash.
**Epiphora**   Watering eye.
**Episcleritis**   Inflammation of the episcleral vessels.
**Evisceration**   Removal of the contents of the eyeball, leaving the sclera intact.
**Excimer laser**   Laser used for corneal surgery, e.g. for correcting refractive errors or removing corneal scars.
**Exenteration**   Removal of the contents of the orbit, including the eyeball and lids.
**Exophthalmometer**   Instrument for measuring the degree of protrusion of an eye.
**Exophthalmos**   Protrusion of one or both eyes – usually refers to that caused by thyroid eye disease.

**Field of vision**   The entire area that can be seen without moving the eye.
**Fields of gaze**   The different areas that can be seen when moving the eye in all directions.
**Fixation**   The eyes are fixed on an object centrally at a chosen distance.

**Floaters**  Small, dark particles in the vitreous.
**Fundus**  Posterior aspect of the retina including the optic disc and the macula.
**Fusion**  Coordinating the images seen by both eyes into a single image.

**Glaucoma**  Increased intra-ocular pressure sufficient to damage vision.
**Gonioscope**  A contact lens mirror used to view the anterior chamber angle.
**Guttae (G.)**  Eyedrops.

**Hemianopia**  Half-vision – unilateral or bilateral.
**Heterochromia**  Different coloured irises in one person.
**Hordeolum** – internal  See Chalazion.
            – external  See Stye.
**Hypermetropia**  Long sight.
**Hyphaema**  Blood in the anterior chamber.
**Hypopyon**  Pus in the anterior chamber.

**Injection**  Degree of redness of the conjunctiva.
**Interpupillary distance (IPD)**  The distance between the two pupils.
**Interstitial keratitis**  Inflammation of the cornea due to syphilis.
**Iridectomy**  Removal of a piece of the iris.
**Iridodialysis**  Severance of the iris from the ciliary body.
**Iridodonesis**  Quivering of iris following intra-capsular cataract extraction.
**Iridotomy**  A hole in the iris, usually performed by the laser beam.
**Iris bombe**  Bulging forward of the iris.
**Iris prolapse**  A section of the iris prolapsing through a wound, either surgical or traumatic.
**Iritis**  Inflammation of the iris
**Ishihara colour plates**  Multicoloured charts for testing colour vision.

**Keratitic precipitates**  Plaques of protein adhered to the corneal endothelium in uveitis.
**Keratitis**  Inflammation of the cornea.
**Keratoconus**  Conical-shaped deformity of the cornea.
**Keratometer**  Instrument for measuring the curvature of the cornea.

**Lacrimation**  Production of tears.
**Lagophthalmos**  Incomplete closure of the eyelids.
**Lamellar graft**  Partial thickness corneal graft.
**Laser**  Light Amplification by Stimulated Emission of Radiation. Energy transmitted as heat.

**Microphthalmos**  Small eyeball.
**Miotic**  Drug that constricts the pupil.
**Mydriatic**  Drug that dilates the pupil.
**Myopia**  Short sight.

**Oculentum (Oc.)**  Eye ointment.
**Operculum**  A semi-circular tear in the retina, covered with a flap of retina.
**Ophthalmia neonatorum**  Severe conjunctivitis of the newborn.

**Ophthalmoplegia**   Paralysis of the extra-ocular muscles.
**Ophthalmoscope**   Instrument for examining the retina.
**Optic axis**   The line through the centre of the optical structures of the eye.

**Palpebral**   Pertaining to the eyelids.
**Pannus**   Neovascularisation of the cornea.
**Panophthalmitis**   Inflammation of the whole eyeball.
**Penetrating graft**   Full-thickness corneal graft.
**Perimeter**   Instrument for measuring the field of vision.
**Peripheral vision/field**   Area of vision outside central field of vision.
**Phacoemulsification**   Removal of cataract by ultrasound, breaking down lens matter prior to it being aspirated.
**Phasing**   Regular frequent measurements of intra-ocular pressure over a few days.
**Phlyctenule**   Small vesicle of allergic origin on limbal area of conjunctiva and/or cornea.
**Photophobia**   Sensitivity to light.
**Photopsia**   Sensation of flashing lights.
**Photorefractive keratectomy** (PRK)   Correction of refractive errors using excimer laser.
**Phthisis bulbi**   Shrunken eyeball.
**Pinguecula**   A yellowish overgrowth of conjunctiva.
**Placido's disc**   A disc with alternating black and white rings for reflecting onto the cornea to detect any irregularity in its curvature.
**Presbyopia**   Inability to focus for near sight due to hardening of the lens nucleus after the age of 40 years.
**Preseptal callulitis**   Inflammation of preseptal portion of eyelids.
**Prism**   A triangular-shaped lens used to correct diplopia.
**Proptosis**   Protrusion of the eyeball.
**Pterygium**   A triangular proliferation of conjunctival tissue that can invade the cornea.
**Ptosis**   Drooping eyelid.

**Refraction**   (1) Bending of light rays. (2) Measurement of and correction of refractive errors of the eye.
**Refractive surgery**   Corneal surgery to correct refractive errors.
**Retinal detachment**   Separation of the epithelial layer of the retina from its neural layers.
**Retinitis pigmentosa**   A hereditary degeneration of the retina.
**Retinoblastoma**   Highly malignant tumour of the retina in infancy.
**Retinopathy**   Non-inflammatory disease of the retina.
**Retinopathy of prematurity**   A vasoproliferative retinopathy occurring in premature infants.
**Retinoscope**   Instrument for objective assessment of refractive errors.
**Retrobulbar**   Behind the eyeball.
**Retropunctal cautery**   Cautery applied behind the punctum to cause fibrosis and inturning of the lower lid.
**Rhodopsin**   Light-sensitive pigment of the rods in the retina – 'visual purple'.
**Rodding of fornices**   Passing a glass rod in either fornix.

**Rubeosis irides**  Neovascularisation of the iris.

**Scleritis**  Inflammation of the sclera.
**Scleromalacia**  Degeneration of the sclera.
**Scotoma**  An area of visual loss in the visual field.
**Seidel test**  A test to ascertain leakage of aqueous through a section or perforative wound using fluorescein drops.
**Sjögren's syndrome**  Syndrome comprising arthritis, dry eyes, dysphagia and achlorhydria.
**Snellen chart**  A chart consisting of graded letters, symbols or numbers for testing central vision.
**Squint**  Strabismus – deviation of one eye.
**Staphyloma**  A protrusion of the cornea or sclera.
**Stereopsis**  Perception of depth with binocular vision.
**Stevens–Johnson syndrome**  Acute mucocutaneous vesiculobullous disease.
**Strabismus**  See Squint.
**Stye**  Inflammation of one lash follicle. External hordeolum.
**Superficial punctate keratitis**  Superficial spots of inflammation of the cornea which stain with G. fluorescein.
**Symblephron**  Adhesion of the bulbar and palpebral conjunctiva.
**Sympathetic ophthalmitis**  Severe uveitis in one eye following trauma involving the uvea of the other eye.
**Synaechiae**  Adhesion of the iris: (a) to the lens – posterior synaechiae; (b) to the cornea – anterior synaechiae.

**Tarsorrhaphy**  Suturing together of the eyelids.
**Tear film**  The film of fluid covering the eyeball.
**Tenon's capsule**  Membrane encircling globe from limbus to optic nerve overlying the sclera.
**Tomography**  Computerised scan of the optic disc.
**Tonometer**  Instrument for measuring intra-ocular pressure.
**Topography**  A contour map of the curvature of the cornea.
**Toric contact lens**  Contact lens to correct astigmatism.
**Trachoma**  Potentially blinding infection of the conjunctiva and cornea caused by the TRIC virus.
**Trichiasis**  Ingrowing or inturning of eyelashes.

**Uveitis**  Inflammation of the uveal tract.

**Visual acuity**  Detailed central vision.
**Visual axis**  The line between a point viewed and the macula.
**Visual field**  Area of vision.
**Vitrectomy**  Removal of vitreous.

**Xanthelasma**  Fatty deposits on the eyelids.
**Xerophthalmia**  Lack of Vitamin A resulting in corneal and conjunctival disease.

**Yag laser**  Laser that cuts holes in structures.

# References and Further Reading

Allansmith, M.R., Korb, D.R. & Greiner, J.V. *et al.* (1977) Giant papillary conjunctivitis in contact lens wearers. *American Journal of Ophthalmology*, **83**(5), 697.

Allen, M., Knight, C., Falk, C. & Strong, V. (1992) Effectiveness of a pre-operative teaching program for cataract patients. *Journal of Advanced Nursing*, **17**, 303–309.

Allen, M. & Oberle, K. (1993) Follow-up of day surgery cataract patients. *Journal of Ophthalmic Nursing and Technology*, **12**(5), 211–16.

Anderson, C. (1995) Combined topical and subconjuctival anaesthesia in cataract surgery. *Ophthalmic Surgery*, **26**(3), 205–208.

Anon (1995) Focus – The cornea–plastic unit. *Eye News*, **1**(2), 20–21.

Barker, B. (1985) *Patient Assessment in Psychiatric Nursing*. Croom Helm, London.

Bonner, E., Dowling, S. & Eustace, P. (1994) A survey of blepharitis in pre-operative cataract patients. *European Journal of Implant and Refractive Surgery*, **6**, 87–92.

Brady, K., Scott Atkinson, L., Kilby, L. & Hilary, D. (1995) Cataract surgery and intraocular lens implantation in children. *American Journal of Ophthalmology*, **120**(1), 1–9.

Broadway, D., Grierson, I., O'Brien, C. & Hutchings, R. (1994) Adverse effects of topical antiglaucoma medication. *Archives of Ophthalmology*, **112**, 1437–45.

Bruce, I., McKennel, A. & Walker, E. (1991) *Blind and Partially Sighted Adults in Britain*. The Royal National Institute for the Blind Survey. HMSO, London.

Burnard, P. (1991) Acquiring minimal counselling skills. *Nursing Standard*, **5**(46), 37–9.

Carson, C. & Taylor, H. (1995) Excimer laser treatment for high and extreme myopia. *Archives of Ophthalmology*, **113**, 431–6.

Cochrane, C. (1993) Contact lenses and bacterial infections. *Nursing Standard*, **7**(20), 32–4.

Conway, J. (1994) Reflection – the art and science of nursing and the theory practice gap. *British Journal of Nursing*, **3**(3), 114–18.

Damato, B. (1995) Ten FAQs on the management of uveal melanomas. *Eye News*, **1**(5), 5–7.

Dhilton, B. & Millar, G. (1994) *The Child's Eye. Diagnosis of Ophthalmic Disorders in Children*. Oxford Medical Publications, New York.

The Diabetes Control and Complications Trial Research Group (1995) The effect of intensive diabetes treatment on the progression of diabetic retinopathy in insulin dependent diabetes mellitus. *Archives of Ophthalmology*, **113**, 36–51.

DoH (1989) *A Strategy for Nursing*. Department of Health. HMSO, London.

DoH (1995). *The Patient's Charter*. Department of Health. HMSO, London.

Duker, J. & Tolentino, F. (1991) Retinopathy of prematurity and pediatric retina and vitreous disorders. *Current Opinion in Ophthalmology*, **2**, 690–95.

Dutton, J.J. (1991) *Coralline hydroxyapatite ocular implant. Ophthalmology*, **98**(3), 370–77.

Elder, M.J. (1994) Combined trabeculotomy – trabeculectomy compared with primary trabeculectomy for congenital glaucoma. *British Journal of Ophthalmology*, **78**(10), 745–8.

Engstrom, R. & Holland, G. (1995). Local therapy for cytomegalovirus retinopathy. *American Journal of Ophthalmology*, **120**(3), 376–85.

Gartry, D.S. (1995) Treating myopia with the excimer laser. The present position. *British Medical Journal*, **310**, 979–985.

Jabs, D., Grell, R., Fox, R. & Bartlett, J. (1989) Ocular manifestations of acquired immunodeficiency syndrome. *Ophthalmology*, **96**(7), 1092–99.

Jose, R., Faria de Abreu, J.R., Silva, R. & Cunha-Vaz, J.G. (1994) The blood–retinal barrier in diabetes during pregnancy. *Archives of Ophthalmology*, **112**, 1334–8.

Kanski, J. (1994) *Clinical Ophthalmology*, 4th edn. Butterworth Heinemann, Oxford.

Kirkness, C.M., Adams, G.G., Dilly, P.N. & Lee, J.P. (1995) Botulinum A-induced protective ptosis in corneal disease. *Ophthalmology*, **95**(3), 473–80.

Kirkpatrick, J., Hoh, H. & Cook, S. (1993) No eye pad for corneal abrasions. *Eye*, **7**(5), 468–71.

Kuppens, E., Van Best, J. & Sterk, C. (1995) Is glaucoma associated with an increased risk of cataract? *British Journal of Ophthalmology*, **79**(7), 649–52.

Laske, M., Connel, A. & Schacchat, A. *et al.* (1994) The Barbados eye study, prevalence of open-angle glaucoma. *Archives of Ophthalmology*, **112**, 821–9.

Latham, B., Higgins, L. & Ambrose, P. (1992) Cataract patient's post-operative eye care: development and evaluation of a teaching program. *Australian Journal of Advanced Nursing*, **10**(1), 4–8.

MacLeod-Clarke, J. (1988) Communication – the continuing challenge. *Nursing Times*, **84**(23), 24–7.

McNicholl, C. (1995) Phacoemulsification. *British Journal of Nursing*, **5**(2), 22–24.

Martin, D., Parks, D. & Mellows, S. *et al.* (1994) Treatment of cytomegalovirus retinitis with sustained-release ganciclovir implant. *Archives of Ophthalmology*, **112**, 1531–9.

Menezo, J., Cisneros, A. & Hueso, J. *et al.* 1995 Long-term results of surgical treatment of high myopia with Worst-Fechner intraocular lenses. *Journal of Cataract and Refractive Surgery*, **21**(1), 93–8.

Migdal, C. (1994) Long-term functional outcome after early surgery in open-angle glaucoma. *Ophthalmology*, **101**(9), 1651–6.

Migdal, C. (1995) What is the appropriate treatment for patients with primary open-angle glaucoma: medicine, laser or primary surgery? *Ophthalmic Surgery*, **26**(2), 108–109.

Milburn, M., Baker, M-J. & Gardiner, P. *et al.* (1995) Nursing care that patients value. *British Journal of Nursing*, **4**(18), 1094–8.

O'Conner, S. & Glasper, E.A. (eds) 1995 *Whaley and Wong's Children's Nursing*. Mosby, London.

Osaka, M. & Keltner, J. (1991) Botulinum A toxin (Oculinum) in ophthalmology. *Survey of Ophthalmology*, **36**(1), 28–46.

Ottar, W., Scott, W. & Holgado, S. (1995) Photoscreening for amblyogenic factors. *Journal of Pediatric Ophthalmology and Strabismus*, **32**, 289–95.

Patel, S. & Speath, G. (1995) Compliance in patients prescribed eye drops for glaucoma. *Ophthalmic Surgery*, **26**(3), 233–6.

Pearce, J. (1996) Multifocal intraocular lenses. *Current Opinion in Ophthalmology*, **7**(1), 2–10.

Perry, J.P. & Tullo, A.B. (1996) *Care of the Ophthalmic Patient*, 2nd edn. Chapman and Hall, London.

Potter, P.A. (1994) *Pocket Guide to Health Assessment*. Mosby, London.

Powe, N., Tielsch, J., Schein, O., Luthra, R. & Steinburg, E. (1994) Synthesis of the literature on visual acuity and complications following cataract extraction with intraocular lens implantation. *Archives of Ophthalmology*, **112**, 228–38.

Pratt-Johnson, J. & Tillson, G. (1994) *Management of Strabismus and Amblyopia – A Practical Guide*. Theime Medical Publications Inc., New York.

Ragge, N. & Easty, D. (1990) *Immediate Eye Care*. Wolfe Publications Ltd, England.

Robinson, A. (1994) Research methods: an overview. *Surgical Nurse*, **7**(2), 9–11.

Saude, T. (1992) *Ocular Anatomy*. Blackwell Science, Oxford.

Seal, D. & Hay, J. (1992). Contact lens disinfection and acanthamoeba. Problems and practicalities. *The Pharmaceutical Journal*, **248**, 717–19.

Skuta, G., Beeson, C. & Higginbotham, G. *et al.* (1992) Intraoperative Mytomycin versus post-operative 5-fluorouracil in high-risk glaucoma following surgery. *Ophthalmology*, **99**(1), 438–44.

Stapleton, F. (1992) Microbial keratitis and contact lens wear. *Journal of British Contact Lens Association*, **3**(1), 5–6.

Thomann, U., Meier-Gibbons, F. & Schiper, I. (1995) Therapeutic keratectomy for bullous keratopathy. *British Journal of Ophthalmology*, **79**(4), 335–8.

Tingle, J. (1992) Legal implications of standard setting. *British Journal of Nursing*, **1**(4), 728–31.

Toma, N., Hungerford, J. & Plowman, P. *et al.* (1995) External beam radiotherapy for retinoblastoma 2-lens-sparing technique. *British Journal of Ophthalmology*, **79**(2), 112–17.

UKCC (1992) *The Scope of Professional Practice*. United Kingdom Central Council for Nursing, Midwifery and Health Visiting, London.

Vander, J. (1994) Retinopathy of prematurity: diagnosis and management. *Journal of Ophthalmic Nursing and Technology*, **13**(5), 207–12.

Vaughan, D., Asbury, T. & Riordan-Eva, P. (1995) *General Ophthalmology*, 14th edn. Prentice Hall, London.

Wakelin, S. (1995) Hygiene compliance in contact lens wearers presenting to an ophthalmic casualty department. *The International Journal of Pharmacy Practice*, **3**(2), 97–100.

Wentworth, J., Paterson, C. & Gray, R. (1992) Effects of metalloproteinase inhibitor on established corneal ulcers after an alkali burn. *Investigative Ophthalmology and Visual Sciences*, **33**(7), 2174–9.

Williams, M. (1993) Achieving patient compliance. *Nursing Times*, **89**(13), 50–52.

Yung, C.W., Massicotte, S. & Kuwabara, T. (1994) Argon laser treatment of trichiasis – a clinical and histopathologic evaluation. *Ophthalmic Plastic Reconstructive Surgery*, **10**(2), 130–36.

# Index